UNEXPECTED DIAGNOSIS

UNEXPECTED DIAGNOSIS

PROSTATE CANCER
AND THE
WAKE-UP CALL TO LIVE
HEALTHIER AND HAPPIER

GABE CANALES

A SAVIO REPUBLIC BOOK
An Imprint of Post Hill Press
ISBN: 978-1-64293-839-5
ISBN (eBook): 978-1-64293-840-1

Unexpected Diagnosis:
Prostate Cancer and the Wake-Up Call to Live Healthier and Happier
© 2022 by Gabe Canales
All Rights Reserved

posthillpress.com
New York • Nashville
Published in the United States of America

1   2   3   4   5   6   7   8   9   10

CONTENTS

INTRODUCTION

It was July 2019, and I was driving back to Houston on I-10 from Baton Rouge. It's the time of year you can see heat waves rising from the pavement, and paired with my exhaustion, it made Houston a mirage in the distance. I was on the end leg of a seven-week tour through America to kick off Men's Health Month, raising awareness for prostate cancer, men's health issues, and urging men to take action.

Over those seven weeks in the summer of 2019, I had real, deep talks with men in rural, suburban, and urban communities, men of all races and socioeconomic backgrounds, across the country. We spoke about the complex challenges they were facing personally with their physical and mental health. I met with urologists, physicians, prostate cancer patients, men's health advocates, cancer survivors, lifestyle medicine experts, experts in minority health, and journalists.

I wanted to better understand what men could do to get out in front of prostate cancer, why men in America are dying prematurely, and most importantly, what's holding us back from taking action earlier in life.

The experiences I had over almost 9,000 miles of that road trip, along with the lessons learned from my own surprise diagnosis with prostate cancer ten years ago at the age of thirty-five, form the basis for this book.

My goal in sharing my story is to motivate and inspire you to take small action steps now that could save your life or save your loved ones from needless suffering. By sharing my background and lifestyle before my diagnosis, along with the insights I gained from talking with health experts over the past ten years, it becomes clear that diet and lifestyle quality is directly connected to lifespan.

I've had to fight for my health and happiness, and I know it's not always easy to make changes. For me, it's a daily responsibility. I hope to inspire you to make a commitment and stick with it.

Prostate cancer is one of the most common cancers in American men. Many people think of it as an old man's disease. We see many public health campaigns target older men, encouraging them to start discussions with their doctors for prostate cancer screening at age fifty-five. In American men, the median age of diagnosis for prostate cancer is age sixty-six, and the median age of death is eighty.

There's plenty that happens outside the median, though. I was only thirty-five when I was diagnosed with early-stage prostate cancer. It was only caught by accident.

I had no symptoms and no family history of prostate cancer—or any cancer. So why? Why me? What led to this diagnosis? Why did I have prostate cancer at age thirty-five? I had a million questions, and I needed answers.

The following years took me through a deep dive into men's health issues. I discovered so many issues were interconnected, and they all shared a common thread—they could be prevented.

I made the time and gained access to experts and innovators in the health and wellness field. I formed a nonprofit and advocacy foundation to educate men and their families on starting preventative health measures young. What I learned, I wanted to share. Before my diagnosis, I hadn't heard these things at all—the information just wasn't out there.

How many hundreds of thousands of men—perhaps millions—had the same condition? How many American men are walking around, living life, not knowing they have prostate cancer? How many men would take action now if they knew it could reduce their risk and save their lives?

I share my story in this book for those men.

CHAPTER ONE

YOU HAVE CANCER

My phone was ringing as I pulled into my driveway. No time to check it. I had been stuck in traffic due to road construction for over an hour and was running late to meet the trainer at Lifetime Fitness.

As I exited my car, my dogs were frantically barking at the lawn guys behind me using their loud leaf blowers. The noise continued as I entered the house with the TV in the den blasting, still on from the morning when I was rushing out of the house. The radio was also on in my bedroom. My mobile continued to ring and so did my landline.

I was hurriedly changing, anxious to get back on the road. The late-afternoon rush hour sucks, and I know traffic will be a crawl driving the five miles to the gym.

I have my gym bag and water bottle, but now I can't find my keys. I've misplaced my keys. Are you kidding me? Did I leave them in the door? I'm now searching the house for my keys while wolfing down a fast food burger I picked up earlier and chugging a high-caffeine, herbal energy drink—my daily pre-workout ritual to counter my nightly four hours of sleep.

It's chaos, but this is my everyday life. I live in stress mode.

I found my keys, got my gym bag, and, with one foot out the door, the phone rang again. I looked down. It's my urologist. My results? I expected a quick phone call, validating my prostate biopsy results showed nothing. It was all a waste of time, and my dad was right; they were "just looking to bill the insurance company." I paused for a second to take the call.

1

My urologist was to the point, "I have some good news and some bad news. First, the bad news, you have cancer."

"Wait, what?" What did I just hear?

I froze.

"The good news is you'll be fine. It's…." His voice faded.

The noise all around me stopped.

"You have cancer."

I stepped back into the house. I leaned against the kitchen wall and crouched down on the floor.

I know it sounds dramatic, but that's what happened. That's how I reacted.

I was stunned. My inner voice echoed loud in my head echoed, "Am I going to die?"

Until I said it out loud, "AM I GOING TO DIE?"

I felt my chest tighten and my breathing became shallow. I was full of fear. I was scared.

I HAD CANCER. Three words I never imagined hearing.

I sat on the floor until nighttime. It was the first time, as long as I could remember, I was still.

Perplexed, I asked myself, "How could I be diagnosed with prostate cancer?"

Prostate cancer didn't run in my family. Isn't cancer genetic? My parents never had cancer, neither had my grandparents, aunts, uncles, and cousins. How could I have cancer? It didn't make sense to me. I thought cancer was unluckily passed down from one generation to the next. There must be a mistake.

I was thirty-five years old and diagnosed with prostate cancer. Just what the hell is prostate cancer? I had no clue. Should I have known? Why didn't I know?

Months earlier, I scheduled an annual physical. I use the term "annual" loosely—I hadn't had a physical since high school, and I didn't go to the doctor unless it was necessary.

I needed answers. I was tired but not sleeping well, and it took me a pretty good amount of coffee, energy drinks, and Diet Coke to get through the day. Two pots of coffee by noon, Diet Cokes, and energy drinks the rest of the day. It didn't dawn on me that four hours of sleep wasn't enough and could affect my health. I got through college with many all-nighters and on very little sleep.

When I scheduled the physical, I expected that the physician would write me a prescription for pills for whatever was causing my sluggishness and inability to get sound sleep.

You see, I wasn't avoiding the doctor; it's just that I viewed medicine as transactional. If I had a "medical issue," I would tell my doctor, and he or she would quickly write me a prescription. Antibiotics for a sinus infection, topical steroid for my seborrheic dermatitis (severe dandruff on my scalp), or pills for when I told the doctor I felt anxious.

When I was sick or complained, I got a pill. The doctor's prescription pad is how I viewed medicine and health care. There were numerous times I would call the doctor and say I was feeling sick, and within an hour, I would have a prescription waiting for me at the pharmacy.

In 1999, while in graduate school, I saw a dermatologist for seborrheic dermatitis, an inflammatory skin condition I had since high school. I complained that I thought I was losing my hair. Could my hair loss be from the seborrheic dermatitis? I had many prescriptions to control it, and everything I took would help temporarily. My dermatologist didn't think it was seborrheic dermatitis. She prescribed a hair loss pill that she said would stop my hair loss and regrow it.

I would take those hair loss pills for the next twenty years. It turns out that after I started, I couldn't stop taking that daily pill because my "regrown hair would fall out." I was never warned about possible side effects from taking those pills, and there would be some severe side effects. Just wait.

I was a busy guy—I didn't schedule an annual physical. I had a business to run. I had an active social life. There were demands on my time that were more pressing. Plus, I thought I took care of myself well. I ran four times a week. I worked out daily. I ate a low-carb, high-protein diet (lots of meat: barbecue and burgers, minus the bun), and I drank a lot of whey protein shakes.

The physical itself took forty-five minutes. Out of all the things I scheduled myself to do, I hadn't taken forty-five minutes out of my year for almost eighteen years. I learned I had low testosterone (low T), and my low T could explain my low energy levels. Like everything else, I thought some pills would do the trick. The physician never asked about my diet and lifestyle.

I made an appointment with a prominent urologist at Baylor College of Medicine in Houston, Texas. I had a test that confirmed my low testosterone levels. I was prescribed a topical testosterone gel, not pills, and every morning I rubbed a quarter-size amount of gel on my shoulders.

The benefits exceeded my expectations: an increase in muscle mass, loss of body fat, and an increase in energy. It worked fast! I had no idea rubbing a little gel on my shoulder would make such a drastic difference in how I felt and looked.

The physician assistant called me not long after I started the testosterone gel to let me know about my lab results and PSA. Confused, I asked, "What do you mean? What's a PSA? A public service announcement?" I'm a marketing and PR guy, so that was my frame of reference. He chuckled and said, "No, it's a test for a prostate-specific antigen, and your number is high." He asked me to come back and take a second PSA, just to be sure.

They had run a PSA when they checked my testosterone.

I'd never heard of a "prostate-specific antigen." Truthfully, I didn't know what a prostate did and where it was. That makes me sound pretty ignorant, but it just wasn't the direction of my interest or intellect. I swear, I had an academic scholarship in college, which I partially attributed to keeping through my late-night junk food-fueled cram sessions. And, honestly, I was doing okay without in-depth knowledge about my prostate.

So, I was a little dismissive of the physician assistant's insistence that I go back to take another PSA test. I hung up the phone, promising to get it scheduled, but there wasn't any urgency on my part. Hey, nothing was wrong. I had a prescription for a muscle-building, fat-shredding, energy-enhancing testosterone gel. That was cool for me, and that's all I cared about.

I talked to my dad later that day and told him about the conversation with the PA. He said, "They're just trying to bill the insurance and make more money. You're young and healthy. Don't worry about it. Suck it up! You're fine."

"Suck it up, you're fine," was my dad's typical response when I told him I was sick or had a medical issue. His other response was, "Don't be a wuss!" That's my father. From another era when "men acted like men and didn't complain."

So, I didn't go back to the urologist's office. Why would I? I planned to keep the same schedule and return to the doctor in another eighteen years or so.

That same physician assistant called again and again, though. He was pretty insistent I get another PSA test. He said it could be nothing, or it could be something, and that's why I should get it done.

"Could be something? Like what?"

He said, "Well, it could be prostate cancer. That's what a PSA blood test is primarily used for—to screen for prostate cancer."

"Prostate CANCER?!" That word.

I thought about it, and it seemed like something useful to do just to make sure that I wasn't at risk.

The follow-up PSA blood test result showed an increase in the number, which I hadn't expected. I was informed I would need to get a prostate biopsy.

I was oblivious to what a biopsy would entail and learned a needle would be inserted in my rectum to get samples of my prostate tested for cancer. That's 'samples,' plural, and in my rectum. Just the thought of that shut me down.

"No way!"

The physician assistant and I again engaged in some back and forth over the phone. Because he said the biopsy would be "just a pinch, and you can go back to work," I gave in and booked the procedure during lunch.

That morning, I had to take an enema, and I also couldn't eat anything before the procedure, so I skipped breakfast, and the hunger pangs were intense. I passed a McDonald's on the way and wished I could pull into the drive-through.

When I got to the urologist's office, a nurse took me into a room that looked like a typical patient room with a table. There I met the ultrasound technician that would be conducting the procedure. I took off my clothes, put on a gown, got on a table, and laid on my left side with my knees bent.

The procedure would surpass my worst fears. It was beyond painful, and it wasn't "just a pinch" like I was told. I should have asked more questions when the PA said "just a pinch," knowing they were going to take twelve samples of my prostate.

First, an ultrasound probe was inserted in my rectum, and my anxiety went sky high. I experienced a series of twelve painful extractions ("pinches?") that sounded like loud rubber band snaps, and this was happening inside me while I was wide awake. It was a feeling I had never experienced before. I was regretting every second of it. Due to the intense pain I experienced, the PA said it wasn't typical, and the local anesthesia must not have worked.

For weeks after my prostate biopsy, I bled, pooped, and ejaculated blood. I was told this was normal.

What is a prostate, and what is prostate cancer?

Men of all ages should know this basic information about our bodies.

First, ONLY MEN have prostates.

Prostate is pronounced prä-ˌstāt.

For more than ten years, I've read it spelled prostRate, and pronounced prä-ˌstrāt. That is incorrect.

A prostate is a walnut-sized gland. A gland is an organ that makes fluids or chemicals the body needs.

The prostate is a gland in the male reproductive system.

The prostate lies just below the bladder (the organ that collects and empties urine) and in front of the rectum (the lower part of the intestine). The prostate surrounds part of the urethra (the tube that empties urine from the bladder). The prostate gland makes fluid that is part of the semen.

Prostate cancer begins when cells in the prostate gland start to grow out of control.

Prostate cancer is a disease in which malignant (cancer) cells form in the tissues of the prostate.

Early-stage prostate cancer, what I was diagnosed with in 2010, means that cancer cells are found only in the prostate. Compared with many other cancers, prostate cancer grows slowly. This means that it can take ten to thirty years before a prostate tumor gets big enough to cause symptoms or for doctors to find it. Most men who have prostate cancer will die of something other than prostate cancer.[1]

Prostate cancer is rare in men younger than forty, but the chance of having prostate cancer rises rapidly after age fifty. About six in ten cases of prostate cancer are found in men older than sixty-five.[2]

In the US, 97 percent of all prostate cancers are diagnosed in men fifty years or older.[3]

Prostate cancer is most frequently diagnosed among men aged sixty-five to seventy-four. The median age at diagnosis is sixty-six.[4]

Again, I was diagnosed at age thirty-five with no family history.

The percent of prostate cancer deaths is highest among men aged seventy-five to eighty-four. The median age at death is eighty.[5]

Prostate cancer seems to run in some families, which suggests that in some cases, there may be an inherited or genetic factor. Still, most prostate cancers occur in men without a family history of it.[6]

About 5 to 10 percent of all prostate cancers diagnosed are hereditary, meaning that an increased risk for the disease runs in the family.[7]

Having a father or brother with prostate cancer more than doubles a man's risk of developing this disease. (The risk is higher for men who have a brother with the disease than for those who have a father with it.) The risk is much higher for men with several affected relatives, particularly if their relatives were young when the cancer was found.[8]

Most gene mutations related to prostate cancer seem to develop during a man's life rather than having been inherited.[9]

A man is at an increased risk for getting or dying from prostate cancer if he is African American or has a family history of prostate cancer.[10]

The incidence of prostate cancer is about 80 percent higher in Blacks than in whites for reasons that remain unclear.[11]

In 2010, the year I was diagnosed, the American Cancer Society published its Cancer Facts & Figures:

> In 2010, an estimated 217,730 new cases of prostate cancer will be diagnosed in the US.

In 2010, approximately 32,050 men are expected to die from prostate cancer. Only lung cancer accounts for more cancer deaths in US men.[12]

A decade later:

In 2021, an estimated 248,530 new cases of prostate cancer will be diagnosed in the US.

In 2021, approximately 34,130 men are expected to die from prostate cancer. Only lung cancer accounts for more cancer deaths in US men.[13]

Death rates from prostate cancer among men in the US dropped by 52 percent from 1993 to 2017.[14]

More than 3.3 million prostate cancer survivors are alive today.[15]

Prostate Cancer - Percent of Cases by Stage:[16]

Localized (74%) - What I was diagnosed with.
Confined to Primary Site (Prostate)

Regional (13%)
Spread to Regional Lymph Nodes

Distant (7%)
Cancer Has Metastasized

Unknown (6%)
Unstaged

In general, if the cancer is found only in the part of the body where it started, it is localized (sometimes referred to as stage 1). If it has spread to a different part of the body, the stage is regional or distant. For prostate cancer, 74.3 percent are diagnosed at the local stage. The five-year relative survival for localized prostate cancer is 100.0 percent.[17]

And five-year relative survival:[18]

> Localized (100%)
> Confined to Primary Site
>
> Regional (100%)
> Spread to Regional Lymph Nodes
>
> Distant (30.6%)
> Cancer Has Metastasized
>
> Unknown (85%)

These numbers apply only to the stage of the cancer when it is first diagnosed. They do not apply later if the cancer grows, spreads, or reoccurs after treatment.

These numbers don't take everything into account. Survival rates are grouped based on how far the cancer has spread, but your age and over-all health, test results such as the PSA level and Grade Group of the cancer, how well the cancer responds to treatment, and other factors can also affect your outlook.

The Varying Screening Recommendations

National Comprehensive Cancer Network® (NCCN®)—a not-for-profit alliance of thirty leading cancer centers devoted to patient care, research, and education.

> "The 2021 NCCN Guidelines for Prostate Cancer Early Detection provide recommendations for men opting to participate in an early detection program (after receiving the appropriate counseling on the pros and cons). PSA testing is appropriate for average-risk patients aged 45-75 years. Patients who are at higher risk (those of African ancestry, those with germline mutations that increase the

risk for prostate cancer, and those with a suspicious family history) can undergo testing at age 40-75 years."[19]

American Cancer Society

The American Cancer Society (ACS) recommends that men have a chance to make an informed decision with their health care provider about whether to be screened for prostate cancer. The decision should be made after getting information about the uncertainties, risks, and potential benefits of prostate cancer screening. Men should not be screened unless they have received this information. The discussion about screening should take place at:

- Age 50 for men who are at average risk of prostate cancer and are expected to live at least 10 more years.
- Age 45 for men at high risk of developing prostate cancer. This includes African Americans and men who have a first-degree relative (father or brother) diagnosed with prostate cancer at an early age (younger than age 65).
- Age 40 for men at even higher risk (those with more than one first-degree relative who had prostate cancer at an early age).[20]

After this discussion, men who want to be screened should get the prostate-specific antigen (PSA) blood test. The digital rectal exam (DRE) may also be done as a part of screening.

U.S. Preventive Services Task Force (USPSTF)

2018 Recommendation Statement excerpt: Based on a review of the evidence, the Task Force recommends that men aged 55 to 69 years make an individual decision about whether to be screened after a conversation with their clinician about the potential benefits and harms. For men 70 years and older, the potential benefits do not outweigh the expected harms, and these men should not be routinely screened for prostate cancer.[21]

USPSTF does not recommend men under aged 55 get screened for prostate cancer.[22]

American Urological Association (AUA) – Early Detection Of Prostate Cancer (2018)[23]

1. The Panel recommends against PSA screening in men under age 40 years. (Recommendation; Evidence Strength Grade C)
   - In this age group there is a low prevalence of clinically detectable prostate cancer, no evidence demonstrating benefit of screening and likely the same harms of screening as in other age groups.
2. The Panel does not recommend routine screening in men between ages 40 to 54 years at average risk. (Recommendation; Evidence Strength Grade C)
   - For men younger than age 55 years at higher risk, decisions regarding prostate cancer screening should be individualized. Those at higher risk may include men of African American race; and those with a family history of metastatic or lethal adenocarcinomas (e.g., prostate, male and female breast cancer, ovarian, pancreatic) spanning multiple generations, affecting multiple first-degree relatives, and that developed at younger ages.
3. For men ages 55 to 69 years the Panel recognizes that the decision to undergo PSA screening involves weighing the benefits of reducing the rate of metastatic prostate cancer and prevention of prostate cancer death against the known potential harms associated with screening and treatment. For this reason, the Panel strongly recommends shared decision-making for men age 55 to 69 years that are considering PSA screening, and proceeding based on a man's values and preferences. (Standard; Evidence Strength Grade B)
   - The greatest benefit of screening appears to be in men ages 55 to 69 years.

- Multiple approaches subsequent to a PSA test (e.g., urinary and serum biomarkers, imaging, risk calculators) are available for identifying men more likely to harbor a prostate cancer and/or one with an aggressive phenotype. The use of such tools can be considered in men with a suspicious PSA level to inform prostate biopsy decisions.

4. To reduce the harms of screening, a routine screening interval of two years or more may be preferred over annual screening in those men who have participated in shared decision-making and decided on screening. As compared to annual screening, it is expected that screening intervals of two years preserve the majority of the benefits and reduce overdiagnosis and false positives. (Option; Evidence Strength Grade C)

   - Additionally, intervals for rescreening can be individualized by a baseline PSA level.

5. The Panel does not recommend routine PSA screening in men age 70+ years or any man with less than a 10 to 15 year life expectancy. (Recommendation; Evidence Strength Grade C)

   - Some men age 70+ years who are in excellent health may benefit from prostate screening.

CHAPTER TWO

ORIGINS OF UNHEALTHY BEHAVIOR

I was born in Corpus Christi, Texas and raised in Houston, the Energy Capital of the World.

When I was one, my young parents moved from Corpus Christi to Pasadena, a blue-collar suburb of Houston, home to petroleum refineries and pungent air. It's referred to as 'Stinkadena' because of the pollution from the refineries that can burn the eyes and induce a nasty coughing fit.

My mom married my dad when she was nineteen and had me when she was twenty. My dad was twenty-five. They couldn't have been more different. However, they were both raised in large conservative blue-collar families steeped in South Texas Hispanic culture. Where they came from, and how they were raised, men and women had their roles; and when you graduated high school, you moved out, worked full-time, got married, and started a family. There was no talk of college in either of their households.

My dad wasn't ready to settle down. He was a womanizer. My mom had left once before, but he would beg her to take him back. He would tell her that he would change and things would be better. She would always take him back. My mother was shy, naive, passive, and easy to manipulate and control.

My father was deeply insecure. He struggled with addiction and didn't know how to control his emotions. His impulsiveness was detrimental, and my mother and I would bear the brunt of it. We experienced years of abuse. The memories of my early childhood are painful.

Next to my bed was a chalkboard. My father would ask me to write my name on it. I would nervously write out my G-A-B-I-E-L and leave out the R. It happened a lot, and it always resulted in my father erupting, shaking me, hitting me, screaming "R!" in my face. My mother would beg him to calm down, but then he would turn his rage on her.

My father would come home drunk, screaming my mother's name when he walked inside the door. She would take me into the middle bedroom, shaking, wrapping her arms around me, holding me tight to protect me. My dad would find us, rip me away from my mother, drag her out of the room by her hair while she kicked and screamed, and he would beat her. When I close my eyes and think about that time, I can still hear her screams. I used to wet my bed a lot as a kid, and my father would become violent. It was a vicious cycle. I couldn't stop wetting the bed, and the abuse worsened.

Experiencing and witnessing years of abuse all before the age of six unfortunately forms you. It did me.

My mom mustered up the courage and strength to leave my dad. She feared for her life, and the only way he allowed her to leave with me was by telling him it would be temporary, like the other times she temporarily left, but this time would be different. She pulled out the driveway in her maroon Monte Carlo, and we left. I can still see my dad in the driveway waving goodbye. I didn't cry. After years of abuse, my mom drove us from harm to what she hoped would be a better life for us. We moved to a small apartment in Houston, Texas. When my father realized it wasn't a temporary separation, he came to the apartment and assaulted my mother. I still see that incident so clearly. He's hitting her in the kitchen, and she's trying to block his punches while crying. She looked defeated. She fled from the abuse, but it followed her. My father grabbed me and took me with him, but just for the night. He didn't need his kid cramping his style with the ladies for an entire weekend.

I feared my dad and dreaded seeing him on weekends.

A few years later, my mom would marry Richard. He was a positive role model and provided me stability and structure. He became my father figure and the person I looked up to. He was the opposite of my father in temperament and in every way. He was a college graduate, a white-collar professional, an avid reader, and he was nice and didn't scream. He showed me a reality that was opposite from which we came.

My grades were horrible before Richard came into our lives. He wanted better for me and believed it was within reach. I was undisciplined and needed attention and structure, so he became involved. He met with my teacher and principal, checked my homework, was a constant encourager, emphasizing the importance of discipline, studying hard, and achieving good grades, so "you can be something in life." He instilled in me at a young age that I would go to college. He didn't allow me to watch television on weeknights. He pushed me to study and read. His discipline and attention paid off. I went from poor grades to excelling in advanced learning classes. Richard talked to me like an adult. He would discuss politics with me, as well as domestic and world affairs. My world began to expand. I began to believe in myself. He showed me attention and love I hadn't received from my own father.

A few years after my mom and Richard married, we moved out of our small apartment and into a beautiful home with a big backyard in an upper-class neighborhood. Big oak trees lined the manicured lawns and streets, expensive cars parked in the driveways, and the occasional big-grinned wave of a neighbor as you drove by. The homes, neighbors, their lives, were all packaged pretty, but that wasn't my reality. Unfortunately, this time in my childhood was when I began to associate happiness and wealth. My never-dealt-with childhood traumas would be compounded with other traumas experienced in my teens and would manifest into unhealthy behaviors carried into adulthood.

The Way I Ate

During the holidays, the family would gather at my grandmother Zulema's house in South Texas and feast on plates of homemade beef and pork tamales smothered in chili con carne. I remember how much joy my grandmother got from hearing us tell her how delicious they were as we devoured them. I would eat dozens, and she would repeatedly ask, "How are they mi hijo?"

"Delicious, grandma!"

Her smile was huge.

All our family members would reach the "food coma" stage quickly.

As we left my grandmother's house, she would give each family member a tin full of her homemade pan de polvo (Mexican shortbread cookies), Mexican wedding cookies, and fudge. My grandmother would mail me a few tins of cookies throughout the year, just to show she was thinking of me. Preparing and sharing her homemade tamales and cookies were her displays of love, and I received lots of grandma's love.

What we ate was influenced by the culture around us. I didn't grow up eating salads and vegetables with my meals. The furthest I got to vegetables was when my mother would serve fried okra. If Texas made a food pyramid, the base would start with barbecued brisket, ribs and sausage, pork roasts, bacon, fried chicken, and chicken-fried steak with cream gravy and biscuits.

I also came of age in the '80s and early '90s—the age of efficiency. Both my parents worked and couldn't cook every evening. My stepdad taught me to make his go-to snack, fried bologna sandwiches, which included fried bologna and mayonnaise on white bread. To supplement that, I'd add potato chips on the side. And if I was still hungry, the freezer was stocked with Hot Pockets and Totino's frozen pizzas. They didn't buy soda, but there was milk, and I drank a lot of it—usually a gallon every one or two days. Does a body good, just like the commercial said (or so I thought).

Restaurants were a rare treat. Eating at fast food restaurants was even rarer. Food was not only love but also a reward. What could be more rewarding than convenient, cheap, and delicious warm prepared food?

Trauma, Triggers, and Food

When I was fourteen, the years of stability Richard had provided me had been slowly chipped away and then taken out from under me. For years, Richard had been struggling with mental illness, but I didn't know that's what his condition was. I knew nothing about mental illness and mental health. Richard had been going to a psychiatrist, but his mental health worsened, and he was admitted to a psych ward at a Houston hospital. The therapy and cocktail of drugs didn't dent his deepening depression, and he was transferred to in-patient treatment at a mental hospital in Dallas. He was mentally ill, and I didn't understand it. To be close to Richard, my mom moved us from our home in Houston to a tiny apartment in the Dallas suburb of Mesquite, Texas, the "Rodeo Capital of Texas." On my first day as a freshman at North Mesquite High School, I saw more cowboy boots and hats than I had seen in my life.

I was resentful. I hated where we lived, the different culture, the people, where I went to school. I had no friends. I would stay up late staring at the ceiling. I was anxious and internalized a lot. I was embarrassed and filled with shame. I thought no one else's family could be as screwed up as mine. I had an abusive dad I feared and a stepdad who was "crazy." I sought a distraction to get my mind off my shitty reality.

Richard visited us at the apartment for a Saturday. It was my first time to see him since he had been admitted. I told him I wanted to get a job at McDonald's, but I couldn't since I was fourteen. So without hesitation, Richard got a razor, took my Texas ID card, and changed my birth date so I could get that job at McDonald's. I worked all summer during my high school freshman year. In those early teen years, I developed a deep connection to fast food. Weirdly, it was comforting at a time when nothing else was. The high-fat, high-salt combination was as addictive as any other substance.

I had a crazy metabolism, and I could eat two or three burgers, fries, and a milkshake in one sitting, and I would wash it down with a Coke. When I helped close the restaurant on the weekends, the manager would let me take home any extra food sitting on the line. Usually there was quite a bit. I ate McDonald's constantly. I drank more soda than I did water. The more I ate it, the more I craved the high-salt, high fat, high-sugar ultra-processed fast food. Like any addiction, I didn't see the harm in the beginning. I loved it. It didn't affect my weight. I didn't think about the health effects. What fourteen-year-old would? I was also making my own money!

Picking up extra shifts, my schoolwork, and my constant worry had me averaging four to five hours of sleep a night. That would never really change. We lived in Mesquite for a year until Richard checked out of the hospital.

After a year in Mesquite, we moved back to Houston. Richard was released from the hospital, and we tried to assimilate back to "normal" family-work life. But a year later, the man who raised me from six years old would put a gun to his head and pull the trigger. He died by suicide when I was fifteen. The months leading up to his suicide were a circus, but that amount of chaos had become my normal. I had become numb to it. I didn't cry the moment I learned he died by suicide—or at the funeral. I suppressed my emotions, and my anxiety became more acute. I turned to junk food to feel better, and I would. I unhealthily connected my feelings with food.

A few weeks after Richard died, I was walking by a tennis court and pressed my face against a fence to watch people whack tennis balls. The sounds of loud grunts when tennis balls were hit felt like a release of some sort. An older African American man was instructing two players. He saw me watching, and during a break, he asked if I played tennis. I didn't. I had never picked up a racket. I told him my stepdad had just killed himself, and I was just trying to take my mind off things.

What an introduction.

The man was legendary tennis coach John Wilkerson, who took Zina Garrison and Lori McNeil from the inner-city and coached them to international stardom. The next day, John asked me to join him to hit some balls. I did. Each time the ball came at me, I swung and missed. He asked if I played sports. I told him I grew up playing soccer and basketball, but I had to stop when we started moving around for my stepdad.

John asked to speak with my mother, and a few days later, my mom came with me to meet John. After they spoke, I learned John would start giving me tennis lessons a few times a week. Months later, when I was able to actually make contact with a tennis ball and get it across a net, John would let me hit tennis balls for a few minutes with a pro or college player he was working with. Every time I had that opportunity, it boosted my confidence.

John built me up and repeatedly told me I could do anything. He was the closest thing I had to a father figure during that time, giving me lots of encouragement, advice, stories of perseverance, and he instilled in me a hard work ethic. Tennis was an escape from my painful reality. I began to play every day. Even on the days that I was working part-time, John would encourage me to hit tennis balls against a brick wall before or after work.

John gave me lessons throughout the end of my sophomore year, but his travel schedule increased. In a short time, I got better. I enrolled in a tennis academy, practicing hours and hours all summer long and through-out my junior year. A year and a half after picking up a tennis racket, I made the high school varsity tennis team, and our team was top-rated in the state of Texas. We had nationally ranked players on the team, and I was part of that team! I worked out a lot and always felt better sweating it out after a hard practice, but my diet and sleep were terrible. My varsity tennis coach never talked about nutrition or sleep, nor did I get any education in high school about nutrition, lifestyle, and mental health.

I would leave campus to get lunch. When I got a car that summer, my fast food world expanded to Taco Bell, Kentucky Fried Chicken, and Popeyes—all located within a few miles from my high school. Every morning when I got to school, I would get my breakfast from the vend-ing machine, which was comprised of a soda and either a Honey Bun or Funyuns.

When I turned sixteen, my mom asked where I wanted to eat for my birthday. "Wherever you want to go." I told her "Popeyes." Irritated, she repeated, "Wherever you want to go." It was Popeyes. She wasn't a fan of fast food establishments. She brought along her friend and they sat across from me, watching me devour a carton of fried chicken, mashed potatoes with gravy, red beans and rice, Cajun fries, and buttermilk biscuits. They didn't eat. That's how much I craved eating fast food. It was my number one choice for my birthday meal.

My teenage metabolism could best be described as a giant inferno, so I didn't see much happen with my body on my Funyuns and Big Mac-fo-cused diet. I was a gawky kid. I could eat and eat and never gain weight. I wanted to gain muscle but couldn't put on weight for the life of me. But something curious started happening. When my diet began to shift to pre-dominantly fast food, I developed two chronic inflammatory skin diseases; severe acne and seborrheic dermatitis (dandruff). My teenage face looked like it was coated in grease, and I started to develop acne so severe that my doctor prescribed Accutane. (Later, Accutane would become extremely controversial as long-term side effects began to be documented—both physical and mental.)[24]

My acne was gone not long after I began taking the Accutane, but the seborrheic dermatitis would stay with me for decades. I used medicated shampoos prescribed by doctors every day for twenty-five years, topical steroids and creams, and even had radiation on my scalp. The dermatologists I saw prescribed medications, but they never talked about what could be causing it—and there wasn't a mention of side effects either. Still, everything was going well on the surface. I ate until I was full, and I ate whatever sounded good.

I headed off to college at the University of Houston armed with the knowledge that I was lucky to eat what I wanted. As a freshman, I moved into a high-rise dorm that had a Pizza Hut and other fast food restaurants in the lobby, along with a few vending machines. That became my de facto kitchen. Funyuns for breakfast, pizza lunches, late-night cram session candy…. It was brain food, right? I started to add in a few "extras" during college—alcohol and cigarettes became part of my social habits, along with some recreational drug use. Peer pressure is a big thing in college, especially with young men—the more you can drink, the more of a man you are, and the greasier and bigger portions you ate were correlated with not eating "girly" salads or vegetables. So, I drank and smoked and continued to eat fast food and avoided anything green.

In college, I opened up to peer pressure and began binge drinking and taking ecstasy (E). It was a great sensation. Alcohol and E gave me a numbness that took away the gnawing sense of pain I had, and they would give me a lightness and temporary happiness I hadn't felt for a long, long time. I'm not really sure if my party friends were as fun as I remember them being or if it was just the haze of drugs and alcohol. But, always, after we left a bar, we would go to a fast food drive-through or a taqueria and binge on greasy food at 4:00 AM. Everyone I knew told us greasy food would be better for hangovers. Go figure. Pumping your body full of salt, fat, and preservatives on top of ethanol was a decent way to make it worse, not better.

Fueled by Funyuns, alcohol, Ecstasy, greasy tacos, and cigarettes, I had an active social life but even more sleepless nights than I had in high school. I got that same industrious spirit that I had in high school, and I got a job at one of Houston's top radio stations in the Promotions department. I worked a lot and wanted to make a good impression. I started off as an intern and soon became a promotions manager. It gave me responsibilities and a new skill set. It was challenging to manage work and a full class schedule, but I was in charge.

I'd set up promotions at bars, nightclubs, festivals, concerts, and cool events. If there was a music artist in town playing at a venue, I would be there on behalf of the station. I'd be there at nightclubs promoting the station and wouldn't make it home until 3:00 AM. Sometimes, I would stay up and go straight to class.

I loved promotions, but I wanted to learn more about the business side of the music industry. This was a big step. I secured an internship for the senior vice president at Columbia Records, Sony Music in New York City. I packed up, hopped on a plane, and suddenly, I was living in a dorm at Columbia University and catching the subway for a daily commute to 550 Madison Avenue. I felt like I exuded cool. The rules of the internship (and New York City in general) were to "work hard, play hard."

I'd work long hours, stay out late, and attend private parties. There was lots of drinking and drugs. Who needed sleep? I was living in the epicenter of the world. I'd stay out late, get a few hours of sleep, and survive on pizza slices, soda, and so much alcohol.

· I came back to Houston after my Sony internship and got hired as a college marketing representative for Atlantic Records. This was another super cool job in the right era. The late '90s meant you had to buy CDs, and I was promoting artists at record shops, festivals, bars, and clubs. Guerilla marketing was in its heyday, and I was out late, drinking, Taco Bell drive-through for dinner, and I still felt invincible. The naive nature of youth. "Sleep? What's sleep?" I barely slept, but I was getting shit done. I was making moves, and thanks to the alcohol, I was the most social guy in any room.

I leveled up even further for my graduate internship and headed to London to work for CNN. It was a busy newsroom, long days, and I busted my ass so I could make an impression. I was a college guy on a very tight limited budget, and I was eating fast food two to three times a day. When Morgan Spurlock came out with his film *Super Size Me*, it could have been based on my diet in London. I didn't get much sleep at all—life was exciting, and I was always ready to experience more. I hadn't started drinking coffee yet, so I'd have six to eight Coca-Colas a day to get my caffeine fix.

The faster I moved, the less I thought about the things that bothered me. The less I slept, the more I moved and socialized—the more I ENJOYED. The combination of junk food, cigarettes, alcohol, and caffeine, along with work, left me high-strung and anxious.

I was always on to the next thing. After my time in London, I found a great broadcasting job opportunity in Miami. It was 1999, and I was leveraging that offer with others, when I got an opportunity to head up the marketing for a dot-com start-up that had famous, well-known investors. The financial incentives were too hard to turn down, and I decided to put broadcasting on the back burner.

These were the early days of the internet gold rush. But less than a year later, the start-up went under, unsurprisingly, with the dot-com crash. The upside was that I had a chance to pursue my broadcasting dreams again. I circled back to the head of the station in Miami. The broadcast spot was gone. I went back to marketing and headed up the marketing departments for two tech start-ups before they also burned through money and had no more capital.

I took a job running the marketing department for an international sports supplement company that sold protein powders, protein bars, and energy pills. I was twenty-six years old, and my diet habits had finally started to catch up to me. I started gaining weight, and it was noticeable. I was drinking eight to twelve Cokes a day. I wasn't physically large for 6'3", but my body fat percentage was high. Being around the "health" industry, I also developed a skewed view of the ideal male body, not realizing at the time that many men I would meet in the industry were taking steroids. I started working with a nutritionist, which brought me accountability and helped, but I would fall back on my comfort food habits and yo-yo diet for years.

The CEO of the supplement company was a famous former body-builder and had hired me from a strong recommendation. He believed I could learn the industry quickly and would be of value. I was ambitious and didn't disappoint. Around that time, *Men's Health Magazine* named Houston the Fattest City in America, and a coworker and I lobbied members of Houston City Council and the mayor's office to have our boss appointed the City of Houston's first fitness czar, with the belief it would lead to a book deal and other business opportunities. It did.

We had it announced on NBC's *Today Show*. He also secured a book deal, and I worked to secure a meeting with McDonald's corporate office with the hopes they would come out with a healthy menu named after my boss. We flew to Chicago for the meeting, and they rolled out a limited healthy options menu in Houston, but it didn't last long. From a business and strategic standpoint, all of the PR, partnerships, and promotions—the Get Lean Houston campaign, the book deal, and the McDonald's partnership—were all to increase sales of protein powders and supplements.

At the time, Atkins and low-carb diets were all the craze, and I bought into them, eating more burgers with cheese, minus the bun, and supplementing hi-whey protein shakes three to four times a day. Meat! Meat! Meat! Protein! Protein! Protein! When I needed an energy boost, I took the energy pills I was marketing, and back then, they contained the now FDA-banned ephedra, an herbal stimulant that had to be pulled from the market due to numerous reported side effects and deaths.[25]

For four straight years, I consumed a ridiculous amount of whey protein powders. I had read a celebrity interview where he said he would consume six to seven shakes a day to help with his muscular physique, only later to learn he was taking human growth hormone (HGH) and testosterone before a movie role.

In my formative years, I'd set the groundwork for how my body and mind would process stress, loss, and challenges. I celebrated with food. I comforted myself with food. I internalized a lot—I had a short temper and a chip on my shoulder. I prioritized external approval over inner peace. I viewed my body as invincible, and when things went wrong, I sought out quick fixes. I never connected the dots between daily habits and how my mind and body felt.

My grandmother died of a heart attack in 2007, before my prostate cancer diagnosis. At the time of her death, she was obese, had triple bypass surgery the year before, and was found dead from a heart attack. The last time I saw my grandmother, she was eating tamales and fried chicken wings. I didn't know much about health, but I knew the combination of her obesity, heavy breathing, and bad diet weren't good.

My stage was set for a health catastrophe—but at the time, I thought I was doing just fine—the road to cancer was paved with my decades of unhealthy habits.

From my 2013 TED Talk:

> By the time I was 35 years old, I'd had 35 to 40 thousand meals with hormones, antibiotics, pesticides, herbicides, fungicides, larvicides, genetically modified, highly processed. That's not even including the high-salt, high-fat, high-sugar foods.
>
> —Gabe Canales, TEDx Talk Houston, October 12, 2013

CHAPTER THREE

WHAT ARE PEOPLE GOING TO THINK?

I only told a few people about my diagnosis. I didn't immediately share on social media when I learned I had prostate cancer. I was processing it, figuring out my next steps and what it meant for my life.

I also didn't want my clients to know, fearing they would see my cancer diagnosis as a distraction. I couldn't lose clients—my income. Also, I didn't know much about prostate cancer or what my prostate did; and because the prostate is in the rectum, I felt uncomfortable announcing and discussing it.

What were people going to think?

I soon realized lots of men around my age hardly knew anything about their prostates or prostate cancer, which is understandable when pamphlets and websites with information about prostates and prostate cancer use photos of older men with silver hair.

I would soon realize many men diagnosed with prostate cancer—even the guys with the silver hair—didn't like discussing their prostate cancer diagnosis and their feelings at all, especially the men who experienced the treatment side effects of impotence and incontinence. I would receive direct messages and emails asking if I could speak by phone or meet in person. I would hear the shame and embarrassment.

Why? There was fear of what are people going to think?

The hesitation and shame men had in discussing their prostate cancer was the opposite of the women I knew that openly discussed their breast cancer journey. Their willingness to be open led to more awareness, education, and funding for breast cancer research.

After my diagnosis, my inability to manage my anxiety began to grow, and at times, I felt I had no control of my wandering mind and emotions. I felt helpless, and I feared the worst. I experienced long bouts of depression. I wanted to get out of the "woe is me" mentality I was drowning in, and though I had been prescribed antidepressants, I knew they weren't the solution. I had been on a high-dose antidepressant for over a year and felt worse at the end of the year than when I began. The pills alone weren't working. For years, I had been prescribed different pills for my anxiety and depression, but I had never been prescribed counseling.

I hesitated to schedule an appointment. I thought of counseling sessions like tarot card readings, just some bullshit that might help me "feel" better. I also considered it a weakness and a last resort. Decades before, when I was fifteen, I met with a therapist after my stepdad died by suicide. It wasn't a good experience then, and I wasn't a willing participant. I didn't cry at my stepdad's funeral, and my mother thought I was suppressing emotions (she was right). She insisted I see a therapist. But in each of our sessions, my therapist would smoke like a chimney, staring at me while I stared back in silence, waiting for him to say, "Well, that will do it for today." During our last unproductive session, he fell asleep in his chair. I went out to the waiting room to let my mother know he was asleep, and fireworks ensued.

So, that was my frame of reference for "therapy." In the meantime, I took the pills to feel better, but I never did feel better.

I recognized I needed help. I wanted to feel better. I kept experiencing these episodes where my breathing would get shallow, my chest would get tight, and I would feel overwhelmed. It felt like I was losing control. I knew there was something deeper that wasn't right, and my prostate cancer diagnosis was what broke the dam.

I scheduled an appointment with Shannon, a licensed therapist.

Shannon asked why I was there.

I responded, "I want to fix myself. I want to feel better. I feel like I'm losing control."

Shannon barely gave advice. She asked lots of questions and listened. She had me do most of the talking. Each session started with, "How are you feeling?" She would ask how I felt about something and why I felt that way. We talked about the different medical opinions I was receiving, my fears of making the wrong choice, my fears of my business going under, my fear of disappointing my clients, my constant need to stay busy, my relationships, my fear of… what are people going to think?

Each time I would talk about why I felt a certain way, it would always lead to another how and why, and those questions would lead me to an uncomfortable place: my childhood and adolescence. That's not where I wanted to go. I felt that wasn't relevant to my issues of today, and I wasn't interested in paying for an hour of therapy discussing my childhood.

I hate the way I feel when I have no control over what's happening around me.

My issues centered around control. I would soon realize from our sessions that behind my need to control was fear, and under that fear was insecurity about "what are people going to think?" I also began to realize all the insane busyness I kept all those years was to avoid dealing with things that had built up that were never resolved. I began to understand that there was something behind negative thought patterns manifesting unhealthy behaviors.

I shared with Shannon a thirty-day exercise I did right after my diagnosis when I entered a dark space. I had done this exercise years before, and it helped—temporarily. Every morning when I woke up, I would turn to the pad and pen on my nightstand and write down ten things I was thankful for. I would write basic things I was thankful for, like having a roof over my head, having a bed to sleep on, food in my pantry. I would think about those things throughout the day.

The exercise helped me feel better before, and I told Shannon perhaps I should do it again. She encouraged me to do the exercise again—but this time, write the "why" next to each item. "Why was I thankful to have a roof over my head? Why was I thankful to have a bed to sleep on?"

Shannon told me taking care of my mental health needed to be a daily routine, not every few months.

She also encouraged me to journal every day. It could be a paragraph or three pages or twenty. She wanted me to get in the habit of expressing how I felt and why. She wanted me to gain awareness of what would trigger my attacks: my chest tightening, my breathing getting shorter, the feeling of losing control. The purpose of gaining this awareness was to pivot my thoughts and my actions so I wouldn't have my anxiety episodes.

I was encouraged to share these and other challenges with those closest to me.

I resisted and told her that's why I was paying her.

"No one wants to hear my problems, Shannon. I don't want people to think I've got problems."

Shannon told me we all have problems and, "Gabe, you're worried how people are thinking about you. But guess what? A lot of them aren't thinking about you, because they're also worried what people are thinking about them. And you have no control over what others think about. You're wasting energy."

Shannon encouraged me to SHARE.

My response would go back to, "But what are people going to think?"

She said, "What people?"

"You know, people I know!"

I began to realize I worried a lot about what people thought who I didn't really know, who weren't good friends, or, for that matter, weren't my friends.

I worried because I thought everyone I knew socially, with their nice big homes, fancy cars, and seemingly perfect life, had life all figured out and lived with no problems. And because I thought like that, I thought of my messy background and upbringing and parts of my life as something to be hidden.

I received my undergraduate degree at a Catholic University in liberal arts with concentrations in theology and communication. My coursework and interest were in world religions, philosophy, and psychology. I searched for meaning, trying to find answers to a rough childhood and adolescence. Why? I wanted to make sense of my past, but at the same time, I was partying, drinking a lot, and messing around with drugs. Why? Because I didn't want to deal with my past, and I wanted to feel good—be happy.

Not confronting and dealing with painful experiences and traumas manifested into decades of unhealthy habits and unhealthy relationships. My inability to manage my stressors in a healthy way would lead to more unhealthy habits. It was a cycle.

But I kept up appearances and lived a facade that I had my shit together.

I wore that mask for so many years.

Shannon asked me to share happy memories when I was growing up. I couldn't.

Shannon asked me to reflect on times in my adulthood that I felt good about my life. I sat across from her and thought about it for a while.

"When I've helped others."

Serving others gave me a sense of purpose. In my twenties, I started volunteering at homeless shelters, disaster relief efforts, nursing homes, the food bank, and clothing drives. I asked questions. I spoke with people in need. I listened, and I experienced time and again that speaking words of affirmation and letting someone know they were heard brought a smile to someone's face. I became more empathetic.

Shannon's encouragement for me to be more open and share was why I called a reporter and did my first media interview. I wasn't comfortable being in front of a camera, but I saw it as helping others.

It's the same reason I wrote my first article for *The Huffington Post*.

Being more open and sharing was why I started the Journey with Prostate Cancer Facebook page, which today has more than 230,000 followers. (Today, it is known as the Blue Cure Facebook page).

That Facebook page was a manifestation of what I was experiencing. I started posting memes of aspirational, motivational sayings. I deleted some after I posted them, thinking they were "cheesy." What are people going to think?

There were many times I deleted them right after I posted them for fear the people following would think the person posting was "weird for posting self-help quotes." And then there were times I was about to delete but then would read positive comments or receive a direct message thanking me for posting words that lifted them up and got them through a rough day.

While visiting my folks in California, I was sitting on the beach as the sun was setting. I took a photo of the beautiful sunset, and there was a quote I read on my phone:

> Life has knocked me down a few times. It has shown me things I never wanted to see. I have experienced sadness and failures. But one thing is for sure…I always get up!

—Unknown

That quote moved me so much that I put those words over the photo I took and posted it on Facebook. That photo I took with that aspirational saying has 409,000 likes, 21,000 comments, and close to five million shares.

Other quotes I posted that lifted me up reflected what I was feeling, and some garnered hundreds of thousands of shares, likes, and comments.

I realized the quotes I posted that moved me were also moving others. They weren't "cheesy" as I often thought they were as I hesitatingly posted.

"Cheesy" was in my head. A lot was in my head. I received a tremendous amount of positive feedback on comments and a lot of direct messages. Many would share how much pain they were in and needed more positivity.

Men going through prostate cancer, their caregivers, and family members needed HOPE.

Everyone does.

The Journey with Prostate Cancer Facebook page would grow to a community of over 230,000, and the name of the page would change to Blue Cure, the nonprofit organization I started to get guys talking about our lifestyle habits as they relate to the onset, progression, and prevention of prostate cancer. A big part of Blue Cure (my journey) would be to remove the stigma surrounding men discussing prostate cancer and men's mental and physical health challenges. They're all interconnected.

It all started with being encouraged to be more open and to share, and I would continue to evolve and experience some peaks and more valleys than I wanted to. But I would grow through the process and become more resilient.

CHAPTER FOUR

SIX UROLOGISTS, FIVE CANCER CENTERS

After I received the prostate cancer diagnosis, my urologist, Dr. Lip-shultz, referred me to Dr. Kadmon, a urologic surgeon at Baylor College of Medicine.

The surgeon recommended prostatectomy (surgery) to remove my prostate. He said it would most certainly get rid of my localized early-stage prostate cancer.

That's what I wanted to hear! An immediate solution. Then, I asked a few questions.

"What are the side effects?" I asked.

He said post-surgery, I would experience a period of incontinence, a loss of bladder control.

"Hmm, okay." I guess I could deal with it.

I would also experience a period of impotence, the inability to have an erection.

Whoa, hold up! I'm sure the grimace on my face said it all. It was when he made that statement that I asked if there were other options.

He told me because of my young age, getting my prostate removed now would take care of the cancer before it could become aggressive. The side effects would subside over time.

No thirty-five-year-old wants to experience a loss of erections. Let's be clear, no man at any age wants to become impotent! But I accepted that I needed to have surgery to get rid of my cancer.

I was going to have my prostate removed.

When I left the surgeon's office, I received a phone call from my father wanting to know what the doctor said. I told him I was going to schedule surgery. My father still questioned my diagnosis and believed there was a mistake. He urged me to get a second opinion.

"For what?" I questioned. "This surgeon is highly regarded and at a renowned academic medical center."

I didn't want to prolong getting treatment. I was racing against time.

But like most things you initially dismiss from your parents, this turned out to be the best advice. I'm lucky that I decided to get a second opinion.

As I shared with a handful of friends and clients that I was leaning towards surgery but would get a second opinion, I was repeatedly encouraged to make an appointment at MD Anderson Cancer Center. The University of Texas MD Anderson Cancer Center in Houston is the largest cancer center in America. Year after year, it tops the *U.S. News & World Report*'s Best Hospitals rankings for cancer care. Their billboards line Houston freeways, and their television commercials blanket the airwaves. It's the first place most of the people I know would recommend getting cancer treatment, even if they've never been there for treatment.

At MD Anderson Cancer Center, I met with a urologic surgeon, Louis Pisters, MD. I was anticipating Dr. Pisters to agree that surgery would be the best option for me. I didn't expect a different recommendation than what I had heard from urologic surgeon, Dr. Kadmon.

But that's just what happened. Dr. Pisters recommended active surveillance, which would involve quarterly PSA blood tests and annual biopsies. He didn't recommend surgery.

Incredulously I asked, "Are you sure?" My question received a deadpan stare. His response seemed annoyed, like, "How dare you question me?" But his recommendation seemed so bizarre to me. How could I just live knowing there is cancer growing inside me and not act?

Dr. Pisters explained I had been diagnosed with a localized low-grade, low-volume (early-stage) prostate cancer, and it wasn't necessary to have surgery at this point. (What I didn't know at the time? According to the NCI, 74 percent of prostate cancer cases are "localized," confined to Primary Site, and have a 100 percent five-year survival rate.)[26]

Dr. Pisters said that prostate cancer can take years to become aggressive and spread, and that active surveillance would allow us to stay on top of it so that if it should become aggressive, we would then discuss next steps, like surgery.

I met with Dr. Pisters to validate that the surgery Dr. Kadmon recommended is the right course of action. It would get rid of my cancer!

Dr. Pisters's active surveillance recommendation threw a big wrench in what I had already accepted as the correct treatment.

Okay. So now what? What should I do?

I had met with two renowned urologic surgeons who gave me very different opinions on treating my early-stage prostate cancer.

As I drove home, digesting Dr. Pisters's active surveillance recommendation—getting regular PSA blood tests and annual biopsies—the thought of experiencing long-term or permanent erectile dysfunction entered my mind again. But so did dying from prostate cancer.

What Dr. Pisters recommended sounded better, but was it the best thing for me?

I was confused, and I was growing more anxious. A close friend recently diagnosed with terminal cancer was also driving my fear.

I met again with Dr. Lipshultz, the urologist who diagnosed me, and shared my predicament. He didn't advise me one way or the other but again told me I would be fine. He repeated, "You are not going to die!" But I was experiencing anxiety attacks, and I needed to act. I had a ticking time bomb inside me.

Dr. Lipshultz asked if I would consider traveling to New York City to meet with Dr. Peter Scardino, who he considered "the best in the world." Dr. Scardino was chairman of the Department of Urology at Memorial Sloan-Kettering Cancer Center in New York City.

"Best in the world" was what I needed to hear. "Absolutely! When? How soon?"

Dr. Lipshultz made the call to Dr. Scardino, and I scheduled the appointment.

I immediately began to book my trip. Since I was going through the expense and taking time to travel to New York City, I figured I should schedule an appointment with another doctor while in New York City. There had to be another "best in the world" in New York City. Right?

My online searches led me to a news story about the prostate cancer diagnosis of radio personality Don Imus, who was being treated by Aaron Katz, MD, at Columbia-Presbyterian in New York City. Surely a high-profile celebrity would get treated by a premier urologist. Could this be the other doctor to schedule an appointment with? I researched Dr. Katz and discovered he was the founder and director of the Center for Holistic Urology at Columbia University. The term "holistic urology" piqued my interest.

I found that both Drs. Katz and Scardino had written books about prostate cancer, so I ordered both books. I was devouring information wherever I could find it. I was hungry for answers.

My appointment with Dr. Scardino was set, but I had yet to make an appointment with another urologist. I was interested in learning more about Dr. Katz and holistic urology.

The next week, both books arrived in the mail. I was like a kid on Christmas morning, ripping open the package, holding both books in front of me.

As I stared at the cover of Dr. Katz's book, there was a testimonial on the cover:

> "Dr. Katz is one of a new generation of doctors that is seeking to move into a truly integrative and holistic kind of medicine."
>
> —MEHMET OZ, MD[27]

The testimonial by Dr. Oz, who had a new highly acclaimed television talk show and had been a frequent guest on Oprah Winfrey's number one talk show, moved me to book an appointment with Dr. Katz.

Before heading to New York City, I read both *Dr. Peter Scardino's Prostate Book* and Dr. Katz's book, *The Definitive Guide to Prostate Cancer*.

Dr. Scardino's book caught my attention by introducing topics and correlations I hadn't considered. He used terms like "prevention," "lifestyle," "diet," and "exposure to toxins."

For decades, I had eaten a "Western diet" of pizzas, burgers, and fries, and I wasn't familiar with a Japanese "soy-rich diet." I didn't even know what tofu was and had never tried it.

Since my mid-twenties, I had been struggling with my weight, seeking help from a nutritionist. He termed my up and down struggle "yo-yo dieting." I fluctuated with being overweight, obese, and then I would achieve low body fat, and then regress to bad habits. My nutrition goals were purely for aesthetics.

I met with my nutritionist before I visited New York, and though I didn't look like what many would consider "obese," my body fat percentage taken with calipers revealed I was obese. My nutritionist said I was "skinny fat," though I wasn't really skinny.

Both of these books were eye-opening and mind-blowing. Up to that time, I hadn't read or heard anything from my physicians about being overweight and prostate cancer progression, integrative therapies, prostate cancer prevention, diet, lifestyle, and exposure to toxins.

What I learned from these two books was all new to me.

This line in Dr. Katz's book about some of his patients who "have experienced the benefits of active surveillance, some of whom on repeat biopsy were found to have no cancer" shook me.[28]

Reading both books had a profound effect on me. A light bulb went on. They tapped into a seed that had been planted the year before when I arranged for a client to host a theater screening of the documentary, *Food Inc.*, which examines the "hidden costs of cheap food," arguing "that mass-produced, 'engineered,' low-price foods come with health, social, and environmental costs."

Watching *Food Inc.* was the first time I started thinking about the food I eat and how it's made. But as much as I thought about it, I didn't change my behavior. However, the documentary *Food Inc.* was what I thought of as I was reading Scardino's and Katz's books and learning about how the way we eat influences the onset and progression of prostate cancer. I was connecting dots.

My grandmother had died a few years earlier from a heart attack. She had triple bypass surgery the year before. My uncle, my grandmother's son, died a few years before, also from a heart attack. Both were obese, physically large, and took lots of medications. They both ate high-fat, junk food diets. No vegetables. I have other relatives who died from heart attacks, and I accepted that "heart disease runs in our family."

I didn't know then what I know now, but I knew the way my grandmother ate post bypass surgery couldn't be healthy. I recall her eating fried chicken wings and tamales. I asked her if she should be eating like that, and she said that the doctor had her on pills and that she was fine.

I felt empowered reading there were actions I could take to make a profound difference during my early-stage prostate cancer diagnosis. My habits could slow the progression of my prostate cancer or reverse it.

CHAPTER FIVE

FACEBOOK

I was shocked at how many friends around my age didn't know anything about prostate cancer, what our prostates did, and where our prostates were located. And I thought I was the only one who didn't know! There was a level of shame or discreteness I recognized with my male friends when it came to their questions about prostate cancer. They were all curious, but many would hem and haw when asking questions, and some would only ask questions via text.

After the local Houston CBS news station aired a story about me wanting to raise awareness that prostate cancer isn't just an old man's disease, I had strangers reach out to me. One guy at the gym walked up to me to let me know he saw my story on TV and asked if he needed to get a screening. He was twenty-seven and told me he didn't know anything about prostate cancer and that watching my story concerned him.

I believed a Facebook page would be a powerful tool to reach men around my age, to share my journey, what I was learning about prostate cancer, and answer questions. I could reach my friends that were too shy to ask questions, as well as strangers who could benefit from learning about prostate cancer, their prostates, and act.

I also viewed the Journey with Prostate Cancer Facebook page as a mental health tool for me. I needed connection with others going through the journey, and I needed an outlet. Every morning I would get an email Google news alert on "prostate cancer" news items, and I would curate articles to post. It didn't matter if the story was negative about a drug or treatment. I felt it was important to put as much news and information out there—good, bad, and ugly.

In mid-August, I sent out the following email:

8/17/2010

Dear Friends,

Some of you may know I was recently diagnosed at age 35 with Prostate Cancer, now the most commonly diagnosed cancer among men.

This year an estimated 32,050 American men – dads, brothers, husbands and sons – will lose their lives to prostate cancer.

Many men I speak with, especially in their 20's – 40's, are unfamiliar with Men's Health issues like prostate cancer, testicular cancer, etc…

I have created a 'Journey with Prostate Cancer' Facebook Page and my hope is to help raise awareness, educate, post daily news links and share my own personal discoveries…and I hope to connect others with many great organizations like The Prostate Cancer Foundation, ZERO – The Project to End Prostate Cancer, Movember – highlighting men's health issues – specifically prostate and testicular cancer.

I have met with two oncologists here in Houston's Medical Center and will be in NYC in a few weeks to meet with other leading experts at Memorial Sloan Kettering, Columbia and NYU. I plan on sharing everything with you.

Facebook Page:
http://www.facebook.com/BeatProstateCancer

Thanks Everyone, I appreciate your encouragement and support.

Gabe Canales

Since I owned a marketing company, I also developed social media strategies for my clients to engage their audiences and consumers. I understood the power, reach, and potential of a Facebook page. And this page would be different than my personal Facebook profile, which was limited in reach to just my friends.

Acknowledging the lack of awareness I had about prostate cancer and recognizing a lot of younger men were lacking in the basics, I believed creating a Facebook page with the name "My Journey with Prostate Cancer" would be a powerful interactive medium to connect and engage men with questions and support families going through their journey with prostate cancer.

I didn't find prostate cancer support groups or nonprofits using their Facebook pages in this manner, so I started a page that would help someone like me in my situation.

CHAPTER SIX

YOU DON'T HAVE PROSTATE CANCER

I received a phone call that stopped me cold.

"You don't have cancer." It was the nurse practitioner in Dr. Scardino's office at Memorial Sloan Kettering.

"What? What do you mean?" I literally pulled off the road.

She said they came up with a "different reading than Baylor and MD Anderson," and that I don't have cancer.

A "different reading?" What did that mean?

I don't have cancer?

I was shocked. I wasn't processing what she was telling me.

How?

How could this be?

What are you telling me?

She said their reading of my pathology is one core ASAP, atypical small acinar proliferation.

She said again, "You don't have cancer," but she instructed me to still come to New York City for my appointment for blood work.

Why? I didn't understand why I would still need to go to New York City if they found I didn't have cancer. That made no sense.

I immediately contacted Dr. Lipshultz at Baylor and waited for him to return my call.

I then called my mother and father and told them the news. They were also stunned, baffled, questioning how could I have received a cancer diagnosis in the first place? My mom asked a few times if I was pulling her leg.

I couldn't believe it either. I spent every day of the last five months anxious, worrying about my prostate cancer. I had become depressed, more anxious than my usually anxious state, consumed with this silent cancer inside me.

The news was starting to sink in that I didn't have cancer. I allowed myself a half-smile. I was processing it.

Hours later, I received the call back from Dr. Lipshultz, and I told him, "I don't have cancer!" informing him of the phone call I received. He stopped me, "YOU DO HAVE CANCER. I don't know what they're talking about. I'm going to make some calls."

It was a roller coaster of emotions I was experiencing. I was irritated. I was growing angry.

Did I or did I not have cancer?

Dr. Lipshultz said I did and I shouldn't have been told I didn't. He told me to continue with my scheduled appointment at Dr. Scardino's office in New York.

I was beginning to disbelieve my sanity.

New York City

Since my prostate cancer diagnosis in March, my subsequent PSA blood tests had been persistently elevated, and a PSA at Memorial Sloan Kettering would show the same. This was concerning.

Dr. Scardino ordered an endorectal MRI. I didn't have this imaging procedure in Houston, and it was explained the MRI using an endorectal coil would provide detail on my cancer. How? The endorectal coil, a thin wire covered with a latex balloon, would be placed into my rectum during the MRI scan. "After insertion, the doctor inflates the circular balloon that sits around the coil and holds it in place during the exam. When the exam is complete, the doctor deflates the balloon and removes the coil."

The preparation included not eating the evening before and the morning of the MRI. I was also required to use a Fleet enema to cleanse out my bowels to ensure more accuracy. The morning of the MRI, my anxiety was high. The thought of having a rod and a balloon inserted in my rectum for a period of time while in a claustrophobic MRI machine was stressful. So, I was told I needed to make sure I was completely cleansed. I hated using the Fleet enema, an incredibly uncomfortable experience, inserting a tube and releasing 4.5 oz of liquid, holding it for one to five minutes till there's a strong urge to have a bowel movement. The "urge" never left that morning. From the time I left my hotel room, during the taxi ride up to Memorial Sloan Kettering, to going up the elevator to Dr. Scardino's office, I continued to have the "urge." And I feared I would lose control and shit my pants, even though there was nothing else to shit.

The MRI with an endorectal coil up my rectum was unbearable. It was a new level of vulnerability I would experience. I was thinking, "God, this sucks!" I was wide awake, and a tech was inserting an "antenna" in my rectum, a balloon was inflating inside me, and I was experiencing an uncomfortable pressure inside my body. The inflation remained throughout the scan, and I was praying it didn't overinflate. I had to remain still, in a slender MRI tube, known as a "bore," while being subjected to the loud banging noises of the machine doing its work.

I was mentally exhausted, physically hungry, wanting it all to end.

My visit with Dr. Scardino revealed no prominent lesion in the MRI scan, and though he was concerned that my PSA was unusually high for the size of my prostate and for my age, he had no explanation for it. He said it could be simply an inherent feature of my prostate, or it may signal a larger more serious cancer.

Most pressing for me was to find out if I had cancer. Just the week before, Dr. Scardino's nurse practitioner had called to tell me I didn't have cancer, and my urologist, Dr. Lipshultz, had pushed back, telling me I did.

Did I have cancer?!

I asked Dr. Scardino. He was considering my persistently high PSA levels and that my twelve-core needle biopsy had been read by two pathologists at Baylor College of Medicine and at Methodist Hospital as a Gleason 3+3=6 adenocarcinoma of the prostate, 0.5 mm in the right apex.

But then what about his pathologist at Memorial Sloan Kettering who said I did not have cancer?

Dr. Scardino didn't recommend active treatment like surgery and suggested in the coming months to have a repeat needle biopsy to rule out a large anterior tumor.

I asked him about diet, referencing his book. He hadn't asked me about my diet. He stressed the importance of being at a healthy weight and eating vegetables and less red meat. That was about it.

I was expecting more clarity from my visit, but it's what I got. No need to rush into surgery or radiation, but do get a repeat biopsy in the coming months.

On to the next appointment....

At Columbia University Medical Center, I met Dr. Katz, who had established the Center for Holistic Urology. He would be the fifth urologist I would meet about my prostate cancer diagnosis.

This would be a completely different experience than my visits with the other doctors.

My PCA3 test showed "prostatic cells were not detected in sufficient quantity for accurate analysis."

Sigh. This seemed like good news. Do I have prostate cancer?

Dr. Katz referenced my consistent high PSA levels and the biopsy report read by two pathologists which showed a low-grade prostate cancer.

He spent sixty minutes of face-to-face time with me in his office, and his first question was, "What is your diet?"

"My diet? I'm from Texas. I'm a meat and potatoes guy!"

He asked, "What does that mean?"

I ate out most meals, twice a day, and because I was always on the go, I ate a lot of fast food. Some of my clients were restaurateurs, and I also ate at their establishments frequently.

"I eat brisket, barbecue, chicken-fried steak, beef fajitas, hamburgers—lots of hamburgers, but mostly without the bun, breakfast tacos with sausage and egg."

With a puzzled look, he responded, "What about vegetables?"

"I love French fries! Tater tots, mashed potatoes...."

Dr. Katz, "Green vegetables? Salads?"

I smiled and proudly proclaimed, "I don't eat them! I don't have a taste for them!"

I said it like I expected a pat on the back and for him to shout, "Right on! You go, Gabe!!"

I didn't grow up eating vegetables, and on the rare occasion they were offered, I didn't eat them. I didn't understand any benefit to them. In other words, I did not comprehend the health benefits of vegetables, or any plant foods.

Dr. Katz also asked about other lifestyle habits, how often I drank alcohol, how I managed stress, how much I slept, how often I exercised.

I was overweight, and he stressed the importance of me losing weight and changing my diet.

Dr. Katz recommended active holistic surveillance, which involved blood tests and an annual biopsy, the difference being the holistic part of the active surveillance. I would need to drastically alter my diet and lifestyle. The changes he recommended to my diet included removing red meat, dairy, fast food, sweets, and adding wild salmon and a lot of vegetables to my meals, with an emphasis on cruciferous vegetables.

Recalling the documentaries that I had watched on our food and how our food is grown, I wanted his thoughts on a statement I heard in one of the documentaries I watched. I asked him, "Are all the hormones, antibiotics, pesticides, herbicides, and fungicides in our foods contributing to rising cancer rates?"

He answered, "Yes."

"Will changing my diet and following your other recommendations make a difference?"

"Yes."

"Can I slow the progression of my prostate cancer?"

"Yes."

"Can I reverse my early-stage prostate cancer?"

"Yes."

I smiled and just stared at him.

I desperately wanted to believe him. I was apprehensive.

I wondered why the other urologists I visited didn't encourage me to change my diet. None of them asked what I ate.

Dr. Katz was passionate and spoke authoritatively.

I had visited four renowned doctors before Dr. Katz, and none asked me, "What's your diet? This is what I recommend you eat, and this is what you should stop eating to slow the progression of your prostate cancer."

The dietary and lifestyle recommendations Dr. Katz provided me gave me hope and offered me something I felt I had no control over. I liked that. I still wasn't 100 percent a believer, but the needle had moved.

When I got back to Houston, I was set on making changes. I knew it wouldn't be easy, but I had to take steps to change.

I purchased a high-powered juicer, took a trip to the grocery store, and bought a cart full of vegetables. Dr. Katz didn't tell me to juice, but I hated the thought of eating vegetables. I just didn't like the taste and believed gulping them down would be easier, and it was.

I became a juicing machine, juicing every green vegetable I could get my hands on—kale, spinach, cilantro, jalapeno, cucumber, bell pepper. I would juice two, three, or four times a day, and every time I chugged a glass down, I believed it was having a positive effect on my health.

I began to recognize I was not craving my Diet Cokes as much throughout the day, I was feeling more energetic, and I wasn't craving "sweet" drinks or snacks as much as I had before. My palate was changing, and I was slowly gaining an appreciation for the earthy taste of vegetables.

I was becoming more conscious of the food I was putting in my body, and I was sticking with it! But there would be bumps along the way, many stops and starts, and I would have to learn how to navigate my triggers.

I hated the smell of salmon, and I didn't look forward to eating it. But I began buying wild salmon, and the grocer would add whatever spices I wanted and steam it for free. I slowly replaced one of my two or three servings a day of red meat or pork and tried to eat wild salmon once a day.

I made a concerted effort to eat less beef, pork (and this was hard because I loved crispy bacon with everything), and fried foods, but I wasn't perfect. I did have the determination and knew that modifying my behavior started by making small changes. I had to start somewhere, and my motivation was the cancer inside me.

CHAPTER SEVEN

THE "SUMMIT TO END PROSTATE CANCER" IN WASHINGTON, DC

I hadn't met any men around my age going through prostate cancer. I became curious if there were support groups for guys like me, so I searched online. I found a few nonprofit organizations: the Prostate Cancer Foundation, Movember, and ZERO—The End of Prostate Cancer. I hadn't heard of any of them, but again, I was unfamiliar with prostate cancer months before.

I contacted each organization and inquired about any kind of social support with men in Houston. I was curious if there were men my age with prostate cancer in Houston they could put me in touch with. Up to that point, most of the men I learned of with prostate cancer were in their sixties, seventies, and eighties. There wasn't a prostate cancer social support group in Houston for men around my age.

A representative at ZERO invited me to a "Summit to End Prostate Cancer" in Washington, DC. I had only been back a week from New York City, and the summit was a week away. I accepted the invitation and flew out to DC. I knew the summit would focus "on effective strategies for increasing the federal investment in prostate cancer research, [promote] community involvement and advocacy for prostate cancer awareness and education, and [give] attendees an opportunity to speak with their elected officials about these issues."[29]

I wasn't sure what to expect, but I was looking forward to helping however I could to increase federal investment for prostate cancer research and to speak to my elected officials.

I also wanted answers:

When will we have a cure?

How come younger men like me don't know about prostate cancer?

Tell me more about diet and lifestyle and the role it plays in the onset and progression of prostate cancer.

The evening I arrived in DC, I attended a reception in one of the Senate buildings where I met other prostate cancer patients and survivors who had come from various parts of America. They looked much older than me, like my grandfather, and some looked very ill.

As I shook hands and introduced myself, sharing I had been diagnosed months earlier at age thirty-five with early-stage prostate cancer, I was met with stares of shock and surprise.

I felt kind of guilty saying out loud that I too had prostate cancer when I wasn't going through treatment, and I didn't look like the other patients and survivors in attendance.

I was considerably younger, and I looked it. I didn't look sick. I thought I looked healthy. But my younger age and how I looked didn't take away from how I felt. The mental and emotional acrobatics I had been living every day for six months could not be discounted.

At the reception, I saw Nancy Pelosi, the Speaker of the House of Representatives, and Senator John Kerry. This summit was a big deal. It certainly drew high-powered elected officials.

I joined a few of the attendees for dinner at The Monocle on Capitol Hill. One of the people at the table said Representative John Boehner, who was known to be the next Speaker of the House, was sitting at the bar. I'm sure he wanted to be left alone, but I was attending the summit to advocate for more federal funding for prostate cancer research, so I got up to introduce myself to let him know why I was in town.

I wanted him to hear my story, know my age, so he would know prostate cancer is not just an old man's disease. My hope was to make a connection and build a relationship. I owned a PR company, and it was part of my DNA to seek out a decision-maker and cultivate a relationship. In my mind, no one is "too big" or "too important" to approach and have a discussion. "Life is just relationships, and the rest is just details;" I lived by that saying, and that's how I viewed people and relationships.

Representative Boehner was surrounded by security. I approached one of the agents and told him why I wanted to introduce myself to Representative Boehner. He turned to Mr. Boehner, whose back was to me, then turned back and nodded to me that it was okay to approach him. As I walked towards him, Representative Boehner turned to make eye contact. His eyes were bloodshot and glassy. I extended my hand, introduced myself, and told him I was in town for a prostate cancer summit; and before I could continue, he jabbed his index finger in the air and shouted, "prostate cancer," motioning a digital rectal exam (DRE). I nervously laughed. He stood up, laughed, slapped my back a few times. He told me to keep up the good fight. We took a photo, and that was that.

All the patients, survivors, and family members who had come from different parts of the country had an opportunity to share their prostate cancer story with their elected officials and discuss more funding for prostate cancer research.

Everyone but me.

I would have met with my congressional representative from Houston, John Culberson, or a member of his staff, but a worker with the summit said the congressman's office never got back with them. I figured there had to be a miscommunication since I was the only patient advocate unable to meet with their local representative. But it wasn't to be. I didn't come all this way to not meet with anyone.

I knew my parents were friends with Congressman Pete Olson (Texas's Twenty-Second Congressional District), and I called them to describe the situation. After a few minutes, my mother called me back and told me Congressman Olson would meet me. I had never met him, and he was incredibly nice to make time for me at a moment's notice and wanted to know about the summit I was attending. I told him about my diagnosis and the reason I was attending the summit, informing him of the patient advocates meeting with their elected officials. He lent a sympathetic ear and then encouraged me to walk directly to Congressman Culberson's office, tell staffers why I was in town, and that I wanted to meet with Congressman Culberson. So I did.

When I got to Congressman Culberson's office and said I was in town for a prostate cancer summit, and I was the only attendee unable to meet with my congressperson or a member of the staff, the staff member disappeared and came back minutes later, and said, "Sorry, we can't help you."

What? "Can I just quickly introduce myself to Representative Culberson? Is there another staff member, a chief of staff, or an aide that I can speak with?"

"No."

I'm fighting the good fight! I'm a resident in your district. Why won't you at least shake my hand? I shouldn't have taken it personally, but I did.

I met up with the other patient advocates and listened as they recounted their positive experiences with their congressperson or congressional aides, feeling heard and grateful to have met. I was seething—not at them, but at my representative.

I kept thinking, "The squeaky wheel gets the grease.... How can you make a difference, Gabe?"

While at the Prostate Cancer Summit, the types of food Dr. Katz told me to eat more of were not served, and the food he told me to stay away from was. There were no sessions or speakers discussing prostate cancer prevention, risk reduction, and integrative approaches to treatment or active holistic surveillance, the protocol Dr. Katz put me on. None of the learning sessions covered diet, lifestyle, and the message to share with younger men about prostate cancer. This was a prostate cancer summit, and I was confused.

Most of the patient advocates I met were surprised to hear about the diet and lifestyle counsel I had received from Dr. Katz and that I was on active holistic surveillance. No one had heard the term "active holistic surveillance," and none of them said their doctors discussed integrating diet and lifestyle changes.

Every survivor I met had gone through surgery, radiation, and/or hormone therapy. No one I met was on active surveillance. Perhaps someone was attending who had been on surveillance, but I didn't meet him.

All this led to confusion about what I was learning from my recent visit to New York and my research.

A chance conversation with billionaire Michael Milken, the founder of the Prostate Cancer Foundation, who was also in Washington, DC, gave me some validation about what I had recently learned from Drs. Scardino and Katz. I shared what I had just learned from doctors in New York City: that nutrition and lifestyle modifications could slow the progression of my early-stage prostate cancer. His eyes lit up, and he nodded his head and began to share the power of nutrition, but he was then whisked away by an aide.

On the plane ride back to Houston, the wheels were turning. I kept thinking about the takeaways from the prostate cancer summit. I was grateful to ZERO for putting together the summit, for inviting me to attend and have the opportunity to meet other patient advocates and to learn.

There were breakout sessions, but none on prevention and risk reduction through nutrition and lifestyle and integrative approaches to prostate cancer treatment. It's not a criticism, but I had come to believe there was something BIG about diet and lifestyle that could save men's lives, and the benefits weren't just to prevent and reduce prostate cancer risk.

I was still wondering why a member from the congressional representative's staff wouldn't meet me. I was looking for a way to channel my frustration and make a positive impact.

I leaned into what I knew: media. I had always been behind the scenes getting my clients news coverage, but I believed sharing my story, my experiences, and my thoughts could make an impact. I was nervous about taking the leap and how it would be perceived, but I went for it. I contacted a friend who reported for the CBS affiliate in Houston and pitched a story about my prostate cancer diagnosis at age thirty-five and how I'm an example of it not being just some old man's disease. It was important for him to tell my story to raise awareness with men around my age. He agreed to do a story. It would be my first TV interview.

After the segment aired, the response was immediate. I had many reach out that they had watched my story and wanted to learn more. They had a lot of questions. That's the power of media. I should have expected it. A guy at the gym stopped me and said he saw my story on television and asked if he should get a PSA test. He said he had no family history, but my story made him think about his health beyond just lifting weights, cardio, protein powder, and supplements.

CHAPTER EIGHT

PROSTATE CANCER: NOT JUST AN "OLD MAN'S CANCER"

I wrote and submitted a piece to *The Huffington Post* called "Prostate Cancer: Not Just an Old Man's Cancer," and once it was published, I posted it on social media, asked friends to share it, and emailed it to my contacts. I was sharing my diagnosis and experiences to raise prostate cancer awareness, screenings, and my changes in diet and lifestyle. It was an article for everyone, but I particularly wanted men around my age to read it. I was getting more comfortable with sharing my story.

I received a lot of feedback and questions about the article. It was a good thing.

The Huffington Post told me to submit articles whenever I wanted, and I did. I wanted to change the conversation and encourage men to think and be proactive with their health. Not be reactive.

My online searches led me to the researcher, Lorenzo Cohen, PhD, the director of Integrative Medicine at the University of Texas MD Anderson Cancer Center. I was fascinated to learn that Dr. Cohen conducts research examining the biobehavioral effects of integrative medicine practices aimed at reducing the negative aspects of cancer treatment and improving quality of life. These include studies of meditation, Tibetan yoga, Patanjali-based yoga, Tai chi/Qigong, and other strategies, such as stress management, emotional writing, neurofeedback, and acupuncture.

I reached out to Dr. Cohen's office to schedule a meeting. I wanted to interview him for a piece I would submit to *The Huffington Post*.

We began to correspond via email, and I shared my story and that I had recently visited with an integrative urologist, Aaron Katz, MD, in New York City. After my visit with Dr. Katz, I wanted to learn more about "holistic urology" and "integrative medicine," and that's how I came across Dr. Cohen during my online searches.

Dr. Cohen recommended one thing for me to do: "You must read David Servan-Schreiber's book *Anticancer*."

I immediately went out to purchase *Anticancer: A New Way of Life*, and on the cover was the provocative line: "All of us have cancer cells in our bodies. But not all of us will develop cancer."

That line blew my mind. How many people know "all of us have cancer cells in our bodies, but not all of us will develop cancer?" I didn't know that. I needed to understand what that meant.

I couldn't read *Anticancer* fast enough.

Again, I asked myself why this information wasn't part of the overall cancer conversation—a big part. Specifically, why wasn't it discussed by more urologists? Up to that point, I had met with five renowned urologists, and only one had discussed an integrative approach to slow the progression and possibly reverse my early-stage prostate cancer. None of the prostate cancer patients and survivors I met had heard anything about lifestyle interventions while going through their medical treatment.

Dr. Servan-Schreiber's book was more confirmation for me that I was on the right path. Dr. Cohen emailed me regarding the book, "What we need to focus on is the cumulative data and the data is overwhelming that lifestyle matters—and it continues to grow."

As I continued to learn, I was more determined to share information about the effects of our diet and lifestyle on prostate cancer. It was urgent. The year I was diagnosed, more than 200,000 men would be diagnosed with prostate cancer. Most of those diagnoses would be localized, stage I prostate cancers, and many men would be over-treated, experiencing years or perhaps the rest of their life with issues of incontinence, impotence, and ensuing psychological issues like depression.

After I finished reading *Anticancer,* Dr. Cohen recommended three other researchers for me to learn about: Dean Ornish, MD, "the father of lifestyle medicine" and president and founder of the nonprofit Preventive Medicine Research Institute in Sausalito, California, and a clinical professor of medicine at the University of California, San Francisco; Gordon Saxe, MD, PhD, MPH, director of research, a preventive and integrative medicine physician, and a founding member at the University of California San Diego (UCSD) Center for Integrative Medicine. He is also the medical director of the UCSD Program in Integrative Nutrition and Natural Medicine, the co-developer of the UCSD Natural Healing and Cooking Program, and the director of UCSD's Krupp Endowed Fund for Integrative Medicine Research; and Walter Willett, MD, Dr. PH, professor of epidemiology and nutrition at Harvard T.H. Chan School of Public Health and professor of medicine at Harvard Medical School.

I learned that five years before my diagnosis in 2005, Dr. Ornish had published the first randomized controlled trial showing that the progression of early-stage prostate cancer (what I had) may be slowed, stopped, or perhaps even reversed by making changes in lifestyle like the ones he showed could reverse heart disease in earlier studies. I thought of my grandmother, uncle, and extended family members who died prematurely of heart disease, and how before my diagnosis, I shared similar dietary and lifestyle habits.

Dr. Cohen, and the researchers he recommended I learn about, would have a profound impact on me. I read about them and their research. I watched their interviews and lectures on YouTube. I would spend time with Drs. Cohen, Ornish, and Saxe. What I learned about them and from them, through their books, papers, lectures, our face-to-face conversations and their advice, would influence my life dramatically—personally and professionally.

CHAPTER NINE

OOPS! YOU DO HAVE PROSTATE CANCER!

I received a follow-up call about a month and a half after I received that call on August 27 from Dr. Scardino's nurse practitioner, informing me "you do not have cancer."

I was informed Memorial Sloan Kettering was amending their earlier report. The pathologist stated:

> "Based on the single H&E slide and IHC they sent initially, I only called ASAP with high suspicion for cancer. Now after reviewing 5 additional levels, I think it is diagnostic for cancer on 2 levels that I didn't have. I will amend the report because of this additional material, and the diagnosis will be: 0.5mm (3%) Gleason 336 adenocarcinoma involving 1 core (right apex medial PZ)."[30]

I was glad for the follow-up, but my blood was boiling. The roller coaster of emotions I had experienced over the last seven months was exhausting. I was furious at the call I received on August 27 from Memorial Sloan Kettering telling me I did not have cancer. I wasn't told there was a suspicion for cancer. I was told flat out I did not have cancer. The nurse practitioner told me they "came up with a different reading than Baylor and MD Anderson." That exact conversation with the nurse practitioner is documented in my medical records. Everything is. Until I received this follow-up call, I had held out some hope that there had been a mistake and I didn't have cancer.

I was frustrated and disillusioned with the carelessness. It was a HUGE mistake. I was angry.

I had met with five urologists at four renowned institutions. On the medical front, I was doing as much as I could and had received completely different opinions.

I couldn't control the medical diagnostics and assessments, but I could control how I ate and how I lived.

I would continue learning as much as I could about the role of diet and lifestyle and prostate cancer, seeking out leading experts in integrative urology, lifestyle medicine, environment, and cancer. I continued to share my journey and what I was learning about the lifestyle-cancer connection on social media. I was doing more television, radio, print interviews, and speaking.

I was invited to speak on a panel at the Society of Nuclear Medicine Conference in Palm Springs. I was joined on the panel by Dr. Faina Shtern, president and CEO of the AdMeTech Foundation. She has been a leader in cancer research and education since 1990, when she was appointed as chief of the Diagnostic Imaging Research Branch at the National Cancer Institute and chair and member of multiple NCI- and NIH- and federal government-wide, national and international scientific committees.

Dr. Shtern learned I had seen five urologists at four different institutions. I told her my PSA over the year had gone up and down, which was baffling to me.

She asked if any of my doctors had told me not to ride a bike, lift weights, have sex, or masturbate for at least three days before a PSA. No, I hadn't been told that. She asked if I would be interested in participating in a clinical trial for an MRI-guided biopsy at the National Cancer Institute (NCI) in Bethesda, MD.

Absolutely. I jumped at the opportunity.

My original twelve-core biopsy in March 2010 revealing my prostate cancer diagnosis was a Gleason 6 (3+3)—meaning, there was one core out of twelve that showed cancer. Would this biopsy, just a year later, show my prostate cancer had progressed? I had sought different opinions. I wanted to desperately believe the active holistic surveillance protocol was working. I had worked hard—every day—to choose healthier dietary habits, to stay consistent with exercising, mix up my workout routines, including more cardio. I was taking an integrative approach. What else could I do?

Dr. Peter Pinto would be the sixth urologist I would visit in a little over a year, and the National Cancer Institute (NCI) would be the fifth cancer center.

When I arrived at NCI, I had another PSA blood test. To my shock and dismay, it had gone up to 5.24. Because I was taking finasteride, a daily hair loss drug, I had been told my PSA was double: 10.48! Double? I didn't understand.

The *Journal of Clinical Oncology* states, "Finasteride causes a fall in PSA by approximately 50%, with a further fall over time, depending on presence or absence of cancer. The drug also causes a reduction in prostate volume by 25%. These factors affect interpretation of PSA and could affect interpretation of DRE in men receiving finasteride, thereby altering the decision to perform prostate biopsy and the risk of a diagnosis of prostate cancer."[31]

My head was spinning, my anxiety levels shot up, and I wanted to throw up. I reminded myself I had to go through the procedures and wait for the results.

Dr. Peter Pinto was the urologist leading the trial. We met before the procedure and went over my records and the year I had lived with prostate cancer. I vented for a while about the different opinions I had received, my high PSAs, the fear in the back of my mind about the cancer growing inside me, seeing a close friend of mine pass away earlier in the year from cancer and knowing others back in Houston currently receiving treatment, and finally my hope that changes in my diet and lifestyle had slowed the progression or reversed my early-stage prostate cancer.

As I lay on the table, being wheeled into a room for the procedure, I began to hyperventilate, and my medical team started discussing putting me under. I wouldn't consent. I wanted to be awake, but I was very anxious. All I kept thinking about was the horrific pain and negative experience of my first biopsy, and the very uncomfortable feeling I experienced with the endorectal MRI. That's where my nerves were coming from, the loss of control, and with the biopsy fearing the sounds of each loud snap, an extraction, and the accompanying pain feeling like my insides were imploding.

Fortunately, and to my surprise, the biopsy at NCI was nothing like the one before. I didn't experience pain like I did during the first biopsy.

As expected, after the procedure I urinated blood and had bloody stool. This was normal, and I expected it for at least a few weeks to a month.

Back in Houston, I received a call from Dr. Pinto. That high PSA of 10.48 had been keeping me up, worrying that my prostate cancer had spread.

My first question was, "How bad is it? Am I going to die?"

"No, Gabe."

He said out of the fourteen-core biopsy, there was no cancer.

Hold up. What?

I asked him to repeat it, slowly, and he said it again.

"So does this mean I don't have cancer?"

He paused.

Before he could answer, I asked, "Have my dietary changes worked? Dr. Katz said some men go back after making changes and later biopsies show no cancer."

Dr. Pinto answered my first question and said the first biopsy showed one core out of twelve, and this second biopsy a year later showed zero out of fourteen. Together, that's one out of twenty-six.

He didn't answer my question about my dietary changes.

He knew my diagnosis had consumed me for that first year. He encouraged me to continue the healthy lifestyle habits and to not continue to live in fear. He said something like, "Live your life."

They had also performed high-resolution imaging of my prostate, and combined with my biopsy showing no cancer in any of the samples, it was good news. However, it was just unsettling that my PSA before the biopsy was so high. I had to look at the bright side. At least I wasn't told four core out of fourteen, or a larger number. They saw no cancer in zero out of fourteen samples.

That first year I had met with six urologists at five renowned institutions. I was recommended to have surgery. Then I was told to just monitor it. Another told me I didn't have prostate cancer, only to later tell me that I actually did. Then I was told it's slow-growing and could be fifteen to twenty-five years before I would need to do something about it. That was followed by another doctor telling me diet and lifestyle can slow the progression, and that some patients have had repeat biopsies with no cancer detected. Lastly, another biopsy one year later showed zero out of fourteen cores negative for cancer (but a high PSA).

What an emotional roller coaster ride. During that first year, a close friend would die from cancer, and other friends would be diagnosed with cancer, none with prostate cancer.

I had been to some of the world's best doctors, best institutions. So, what to make of all of it?

The first year, after my diagnosis, I had done a lot of reading. After my meeting with Dr. Katz, I researched a lot on diet and prostate cancer, and overall diet, lifestyle, and cancer.

It had become so clear to me that year that all my family members who had passed away the decade before were all overweight, obese, and had unhealthy dietary and lifestyle habits. Though none of them had died of cancer, I was connecting dots.

My dietary habits had significantly changed, and I recognized the degree of change when I was around members of my family. Their eating habits were just like mine before my diagnosis. I thought about the members of my family who had passed away, and I wondered if they had adopted similar dietary habits; would they still be alive? Could they have prevented or significantly reduced their risk of dying from heart disease, diabetes, and stroke?

Hearing my biopsy results from Dr. Pinto fired me up even more to seek out experts in diet, lifestyle, and prostate cancer, and overall cancer prevention, to learn more. This was my quest. This was my mission, and I would devote my life to help get that message out to millions.

CHAPTER TEN

ERECTIONS AND MAN BOOBS

My fear of surgery for my early-stage prostate cancer was knowing there would be a period I would experience erectile dysfunction. I was never told how long it could last, just that I would regain erectile function.

For the last ten-plus years, I have spoken and corresponded with hundreds of men who shared their anger, frustration, and depression from being impotent. Many men regretted having surgery for early-stage prostate cancer but felt pressured by their spouse or partner to have the "cancer removed."

When I first started posting on the Blue Cure Facebook page about men experiencing erectile dysfunction, I would read comments posted from men proclaiming they had surgery, and everything was working 100 percent!

Some of those same men would later privately share with me they never regained their erectile function. They felt worthless as a partner and thought about suicide.

I became more empathetic when I began to experience the same, and I hadn't had surgery or any other medical treatment.

After my biopsy, I noticed a difference in my erections. They weren't as hard. I was slightly bothered by it but passed it off as stress-related. This continued throughout the year. The next year, after my second biopsy, my erections were getting even less hard. Now I was beginning to get concerned.

Did the biopsies influence my erections?

I began to research online and found there were studies that showed men had experienced erectile dysfunction (ED) after a biopsy. I was angry. I wondered whether I would have still had the procedure if I had known this before.

Yeah, I probably would have still had the biopsy to know if I had prostate cancer.

My blood was boiling. Would my, dare I say, erectile dysfunction, become worse? Would it be permanent?

I spoke with my urologist and was told my ED should resolve, and I was given pills to take before I had sex.

I took the pills a few times, and my face flushed, my eyes felt like they were being stabbed, and I had a headache that lasted hours. How do men have sex like this? My erections were a little firmer, but it wasn't worth it. I shared this with my doctor, and he said all men respond differently and that there were different ED medications for me to try. He loaded me up with a bag of samples. Some I experienced fewer side effects than others. None of them were a panacea. I wanted my erections to be like they were before my biopsy procedures: hard as a rock.

By this time, I had made many friends who were urologists, and I shared my ED concerns with a few. They all agreed it could be from the biopsy, and they also said stress and my age were factors. I was thirty-six at that time, and literally a year before, I was good in that department. Again, I was encouraged to try different medications for erectile dysfunction and was told it's not that big a deal.

But it was to me.

I became aware that erectile dysfunction was a risk factor for heart disease. I was all too familiar with heart disease, which had killed some of my family members. They all ate poorly, so I also considered my diet as a factor, though I was convinced it was the biopsies.

The erectile dysfunction worsened over the next few years, and I got to a point when I couldn't have erections. Since I was a teenager, I would wake up with erections. That's normal. I was no longer waking up with an erection. I couldn't be stimulated to get an erection. My sex drive was there, but the erections just weren't happening. It was affecting me mentally, emotionally, and socially. I felt inadequate to date. I didn't feel like a man. I now fully understood the emotional pain men had been confiding in me. So, so many men were embarrassed to discuss it, and now I was too. I couldn't bring myself to share it with anyone close to me, and I wouldn't share it on social media. I was so embarrassed I didn't even tell Shannon, my therapist. I told Shannon everything else about my life, every dark moment, every pain, but I couldn't share that I was experiencing erectile dysfunction.

My mental state was affecting my healthy intentions.

My weight would fluctuate from two-hundred pounds, up to two-fifteen, then way back up to two-thirty-five. My anxiety and depression were leading me to binge eat. I was no longer eating red meat, dairy, and fast food, but I was compensating with sugar binges, which I absolutely knew wasn't healthy. It was impulsive.

Then, another medical issue would arise.

One day after getting out of the shower, I stared at my reflection in the mirror and noticed something different. My chest looked different. I was lean at that time, and I could see my obliques and definition in my arms and shoulders, but my chest looked different. My left pec looked like a woman's breast. I stared in the mirror for a long time while I gripped my pec. I squeezed my left pec, then my right pec. I felt them both at the same time. I felt below my nipple on my left pec and felt something. I squeezed hard and felt a mass, a hard knot, and smaller knots.

My heart sank.

The first thing I thought of: Cancer.

Fuck!

I was living with early-stage prostate cancer, trying my best to live healthier, experiencing severe erectile dysfunction. I had no social life, I was growing a boob (why was I growing a boob?!?!), and I thought I might have male breast cancer, and I was filled with so much shame. It didn't help at all that I went down a Google rabbit hole for men's breast cancer.

I started journaling again. I began to write what I was grateful for and worked hard to get out of the dark hole. I didn't tell anyone about the knot

I felt in my pec, and I didn't tell Shannon. I tried my best to put on a happy face, but the shame continued to grow, and so did my depression. I didn't feel like a man. There were times I thought of just jumping off the balcony of my eighth-floor apartment.

I focused on my workouts. I lifted weights and did cardio. I was lean again, but I had a man-boob, and I thought I looked like a freak. It affected me to the point I changed my daily routine. When I changed clothes in the gym locker room, I would change my shirt in one of the stalls. I worked out with a towel draped over my left shoulder, covering my pec. I wouldn't take off my shirt at the pool and beach. That's how self-conscious I was. Every night I would squeeze my chest and feel that clumpy mass growing larger behind my nipple.

When I looked at photos from events, I focused on my chest to see if my man-boob was noticeable, if one side of my suit or shirt protruded. I saw that it did. I cropped the photos I was in and wore looser shirts.

I reached out to a urologist buddy of mine, sent him photos of my man-boob, and told him about the lump I felt.

He said it looked like gynecomastia, an "increase in the amount of breast gland tissue in boys or men, caused by an imbalance of the hormones estrogen and testosterone."

He encouraged me to get it checked out, but I waited. I didn't want to find out I had another cancer. The irony, how I had been encouraging men not to delay getting their checkups to catch medical issues early when they're most treatable, and yet, fear drove my decision to avoid the doctor. I get it.

As time passed, I realized whatever it was, the longer I waited, the more it grew, and the worse it could be to treat. I needed to act.

In 2018, I finally visited a highly regarded plastic surgeon at the Texas Medical Center in Houston. The surgeon examined my chest and confirmed I did have gynecomastia on both sides of my chest. One side was more severe than the other. I asked if it was cancer, and he said probably not, but that I would need to have surgery, and the specimens would be sent to a pathologist.

I didn't want to hear I needed surgery. I hoped for a quick fix using creams, gels, or pills. The doctor told me that in my case, I would need surgery.

I asked the surgeon about a disturbing piece of information I had just uncovered. I had read that the hair loss pill I had been taking for nineteen years had a side effect of gynecomastia reported by some men.[32]

Prolonged oral use of finasteride leads to the emergence of sexual disorders including decrease in libido, gynecomastia, erectile dysfunction, ejaculation disorder, orgasm disorders, and mood disturbances.[33]

He asked if I was still taking the pill. I told him I was, and he asked why. I told him it was because I didn't want to lose my hair. He said, "But you have a full head of hair!" I told him that my dermatologist told me nineteen years before that if I stopped taking the pill, the hair that I had regrown would fall out.

Though the physician was a plastic surgeon and in the business of helping patients look and feel better about their appearance, he was bald and just stared at my full head of hair, shook his head, and suggested I stop taking the pill. I asked if he knew if the information I read was true. He couldn't say.

I scheduled the surgery.

That evening, I researched more about the links between the hair loss pill I had been taking and gynecomastia. I found there was a lot more information linking the two, as well as another side effect that caught me by surprise: erectile dysfunction.[34]

I read there were lawsuits all over the world against the drug manufacturer for not warning physicians and consumers about side effects and depressive symptoms.[35]

I couldn't believe it. My dermatologist never mentioned side effects. My urologists knew I took the drug for a solution for my hair loss. He prescribed me a pill to give me erections.

I continued to research. The more I read, the more disturbed I became. I spoke with two buddies about the hair loss pill. Both had receding hairlines, and, on a hunch, I suspected one or both might have taken the pill. Both had, past tense. I couldn't tell them what I was going through yet, but I was asking for their feedback on the drug since I saw it heavily advertised everywhere. They each told me separately they took it and then stopped because of side effects. I probed and asked what kind of side effects and they both said it had affected their erections. One told me he just couldn't get it up. I asked if they had told others. They both said I was the first person they told.

I wondered how many men—especially younger men—bombarded with advertisements for hair loss, ordered the pills, experienced erectile dysfunction, and never told anyone and/or also ordered the pills to help with erections.

My research showed that some of the men who took the hair loss pill experienced erectile dysfunction. After stopping that medication, some regained erectile function, and some never regained function.

The only way for me to know was to stop taking the hair loss pill, and I did. Time would tell.

I arrived at the hospital without any sleep the night before. I was physically and mentally exhausted, but I was ready to have the surgery. I did not want to go under, but I had no choice. Yes, people every day have surgery, and they go under, and they're fine. What can I say? I get nervous.

I was in my patient gown, sitting upright on the bed, being prepped. The anesthesiologist visited, and a few minutes after he left, his assistant came by and told me that in thirty minutes or so, they would wheel me down the hall. She snapped something in the IV. I blinked, woke up, and I had tubes running out from under my armpits, draining blood, with a compression vest around my chest.

For about a week, throughout the day, I emptied the drains safety-pinned to my compression vest. I was draining a lot of blood but was told it wasn't cause for concern. I was curious to see my chest. I would have to wait, due to the compression vest.

At a follow-up appointment, I was told there was no cancer found, and that was a huge relief. It was the best news of the day. The doctor removed the tubes and slowly removed my bandages to examine my chest. I stood up and looked at my chest in the full-length mirror. I didn't like what I saw. My bruised chest looked deformed. The surgeon told me he had to go through both my nipples to remove the glandular tissue, and he said there was a lot on the left side. As I stared at my indented chest and sewn nipples in the mirror. I told him I didn't expect it to look the way it did. I was in shock. He promised me it would look different a year later. It would look like a normal chest. Give it time.

I was off the hair loss pill, and time would tell if I regained my erections and if my hair would quickly fall out as I had been warned. I was just glad to be off that pill. There were numerous studies and recent reports that continued to link the drug to sexual side effects, including reduced volume of ejaculate, decreased libido, erectile dysfunction, enlarged breasts, depression, and suicide.[36]

These were lessons I planned to share from this experience. In due time. I needed to heal, and my focus was on building my mental and physical health.

As I began to recover, I thought about how every health issue I was experiencing was linked to my diet, lifestyle, or a drug I had taken.

That's true for most Americans.

I was fired up. I was motivated to take my advocacy on the road.

CHAPTER ELEVEN

A BLUE CURE

I can't share the lessons I've learned in my prostate cancer journey without talking about Blue Cure, the nonprofit organization I founded as a result of my experiences living with prostate cancer and learning about the influence of diet and lifestyle.

I made the following realizations about myself and men's health in America over the months after my diagnosis:

> Many men in America are overweight. That was me before my diagnosis.

> Many men in America are obese (approaching half). That was me before my diagnosis.

> Most men in America have a lifestyle-driven chronic health condition. That was me before my diagnosis.

> Most men don't schedule an annual physical. That was me before my diagnosis.

> Most men I talked to have low men's health literacy. That was me before my diagnosis.

Most men don't openly discuss their health issues, and most I've spoken to feel shame and stigma discussing mental health challenges. That was me before my diagnosis.

Most men don't understand the link between diet, lifestyle, and disease and cancer. That was me before my diagnosis.

Most men I've talked to have no idea the function of their prostate. That was me before my diagnosis.

Everything I just listed was me before my diagnosis and the men in my family who have died prematurely or are living with a lifestyle-driven chronic health condition.

The realizations were all interconnected. I didn't want others to be like me and find themselves with an unexpected diagnosis with an "old man's cancer" at age thirty-five.

I wanted to do something to keep that from happening. I realized there was a big problem, a severe lack of knowledge and profound shame discussing men's health issues. Why was I, the men in my family, my male friends, and most of the men I met not open to discussing our health issues and scheduling annual checkups?

Through the correspondence I had through the Journey with Prostate Cancer Facebook page, and from the feedback I received after my early media interviews, I recognized a severe lack of men's health and prostate cancer literacy with the men in my family, friends, and acquaintances.

My diagnosis was my wake-up call. Out of fear and uncertainty came a determination to get answers. The more I learned, the more motivated I became to share that knowledge and my experiences. I recognized the power of sharing and how it helps others. I was determined to live an anti-cancer lifestyle and beat early-stage prostate cancer—and stave off heart disease, stroke, and diabetes, which had taken the lives of my loved ones. I wanted to shine a continuous light on the links between lifestyle and prostate cancer, and men's health literacy and prevention.

I believed forming a nonprofit organization would allow me to make that difference. It would open doors for me to speak with more leading medical professionals, researchers, and lifestyle experts. And that would provide the knowledge and additional resources to further my ability to raise awareness about prostate cancer prevention and risk reduction with diet and lifestyle, specifically targeting younger men around my age.

It was about helping others, but I knew the process of starting it and curating and developing content and programs to help others would teach me more than I could imagine in my continuous journey with prostate cancer.

I turned to my friend, Brandon Coleman, a retired successful business and branding strategist, who, years before, counseled me when I started my marketing company and is who I reached out to and sought advice about creating a nonprofit organization. He's in the age range when men more openly get prostate cancer screenings and has an interest in issues surrounding men's health. He's a brilliant and successful strategist and a no-bullshit guy. He would tell me if I was wasting my time trying to do something that's already been done.

We met a few times at a local coffee shop where I articulated my vision to answer the why. What was the need not being met? Why was I doing this? I shared the experiences I had with urologists and the conversations I had with many men. I discussed the severe lack of prostate cancer and men's health literacy. We talked about how unique my story was and how that could be used to draw attention to the issue of prostate cancer and get younger men to be proactive, making lifestyle choices to get out in front of the disease. With my marketing and public relations background and skill set, I knew I could use my voice and talent to make an impact. Brandon agreed.

My friend researched how other prostate cancer nonprofit organizations were reaching men and younger men with the lifestyle message on prostate cancer education and prevention. He acknowledged there was a tremendous opportunity. What I was learning about the link between lifestyle and prostate cancer wasn't widely disseminated in public health campaigns and by prostate cancer nonprofits to men—not to men around my age. This was the opportunity. This is what I would work to change.

We brainstormed for hours, batting around names and logos that would fit my vision for this nonprofit. Brandon came up with the name

"Blue Cure"—"blue" for men, and the double-meaning of "cure" for life-style and prevention and the medical "cure" we all seek. Brandon said Blue Cure is the blue side to the women's pink movement for breast cancer, but that it should be positioned to appeal to women. "They are the key to influencing their husbands, fathers, sons, and brothers."

I wasn't at the point where I was "okay" living with early-stage prostate cancer. Every day I lived with fear, anxiety and struggled with bouts of depression, but I was working through it.

Too many men I had spoken with had "awareness" of the two words prostate cancer but didn't know anything about it, nor the function of their prostate, where it was, the dietary and lifestyle habits that influence prostate cancer initiation and progression, what age to get screened, and that most prostate cancers are not a death sentence.

What I was learning about diet and lifestyle was empowering. That's what I wanted to share with men, and I wanted them to know that now—decades before they get screened and before some are diagnosed with prostate cancer. Just so I'm clear from the beginning, I believed and advocated that part of a healthy lifestyle included getting in the habit of getting an annual physical.

Pharmaceutical Money

Before I publicly shared why I was starting the Blue Cure nonprofit, I called a publicist I had worked with years before on a project. I valued her expertise. She was New York-based, savvy, and the most connected publicist I knew. Her agency represented major brands, celebrities, and media outlets. She could pick up the phone and have a client written about in the *New York Times* or booked on the *Today Show* (as she did for my former boss). I wasn't her client, but she gave me twenty minutes of her time to share what I was doing and why. She wanted to know what was unique about it.

I shared my journey and how adding my voice to the conversation on prostate cancer and men's health issues could change the way some men approach the disease.

She grew excited the more I shared my aspirations to target younger men and promote prevention with lifestyle change.

She interrupted, "Damn it! We just resigned an account (major fashion brand), and I told them to do a blue campaign for men's health! This lifestyle message would have been perfect to introduce to them!"

She explained she saw the need because men in her life were reluctant to be proactive with their health, and prevention was not a message that men were hearing. She urged me to be true to my mission by remaining "pure" and not partnering with companies that didn't align with the vision.

I wasn't expecting what came next. In her thick New York accent, she challenged me, "Don't take fucking pharma money!"

I asked, "Why?" She said Blue Cure should not be perceived as a shill for a drug maker.

"A shill for a drug maker?" What was she talking about?

She continued, "They have the fucking money, but I'm telling you. They will want you to promote their drug, and your message will get lost."

I'm not, nor was I, "anti-pharma." I wasn't advocating for alternative medicine. I believed in science. I was hopeful about drug treatments, but what was missing and urgently needed was a lifestyle message targeting men. There needed to be more information on taking a holistic, whole-body approach for prostate cancer prevention, on people like me on active surveillance (active holistic surveillance), and on how such an approach could improve outcomes for men using medical intervention and reduce the recurrence of the disease.

I hadn't considered how I would raise money to support getting this message out there. I didn't contemplate fundraising events, runs, dinners, etc. That wasn't my priority. The fear of living with cancer and being overcome by it was constantly in my head. That fear and knowing others with terminal cancer compelled me to go forward without considering how I would raise funds to get the message out. I just jumped in and did it. I had to, with what was going on in my head. I felt better believing I was doing something that could help others. The publicist's counsel had an impact on me, and I heeded her words.

My naivete was believing that a simple "Donate" button on a website would be enough. When people learned what made Blue Cure's message unique and necessary to bring about change, people would see the good in that and donate whatever they could to help us get the message out to men of all ages.

I never wanted Blue Cure to be perceived as "bought," and I would learn over the years that "Big Pharma," "Big Food," "Big Soda"—all the Bigs—have big money. Patient advocacy nonprofit groups receive lots of money from pharmaceutical companies.·

Unless an organization has a lot of capital to get the operation off the ground, it can be challenging to get the message out and sustain those efforts when you don't have big funding to support it.

Have you heard of Big Broccoli? Big Tofu?

I didn't think so.

I bring this up because I've been asked why Blue Cure doesn't have pharma banners at our runs, events, buying tables at our events. Pharmaceutical money has enabled a large prostate cancer nonprofit to grow nationwide, which also helps the nonprofit raise money for its programs.

Pharma generates hundreds of billions in annual revenue. In 2019, while I was driving the country on a nationwide men's health tour, I received a call from a representative of a major pharmaceutical company. She wanted to learn more about Blue Cure and discuss ways to partner so they could support our programs. We had a series of calls, and she pointedly said after viewing some of my media interviews she thought I could be anti-pharma. I asked why she thought that and told her there isn't one article I've written nor any media interviews or speeches I've given in the last nine years that were "anti-pharma." The representative asked about a Blue Cure video that showed Richard Nixon signing the Cancer Act of 1971 and stated that over $100 billion had been spent on research and we still didn't have a medical cure.

I told her that was true. The point of the video was while various entities continue to fund billions on research for a medical cure, we should ALSO allocate resources for education on prevention. At the time, various organizations reported that half of cancers and cancer deaths were preventable. She told me I needed to stay away from messaging like that to receive their funding. She asked if I would meet with an executive when I drove through New York. I did.

I met the executive at a vegetarian restaurant in lower Manhattan and dined for a few hours. He previously worked in Congress and was now working for a pharmaceutical giant. He expressed his genuine interest in the uniqueness of my message, that I was Hispanic and had minority outreach campaigns. He told me it would be "easy" to purchase a $10,000 table at a future Lecture Series, and that there was a lot more they could do to support Blue Cure. I asked what was asked for in return for their financial support, and he said nothing, "no strings attached," we just want to support your efforts. As we parted ways, he asked if I would be open to coming back in the future and give a presentation to other members of the company, and I said I would.

When I got back on the road and continued the men's health tour, the representative who set up the original meeting asked me to submit a proposal on why they should support Blue Cure and how they would be acknowledged.

I never did.

Prostate Cancer Nonprofit

The COO of a national prostate cancer nonprofit called me and inquired about hiring me—the services of my marketing company—to develop a marketing and public relations strategy. I was flattered he reached out. I told him I was starting a nonprofit to add a voice to the prostate cancer community, and I couldn't take on any new clients. He expressed surprise with what I was telling him, and I explained the nonprofit would have a strong emphasis on reaching younger men around my age since most guys my age weren't educated about prostate cancer. He encouraged me to reconsider starting the nonprofit and work with their nonprofit instead, letting me know they had an infrastructure in place, they had established donors and corporate support, and it would be very hard for me to start from scratch and grow it nationally. He was sincere, and I recognized their organization had support from the major pharmaceutical companies and thousands of individual donors.

But still, I pushed back that their organization and others had their missions. I was thirty-five with prostate cancer, and I had never heard about any prostate cancer nonprofit before my diagnosis. I explained that guys my age have little to no prostate cancer literacy and that there weren't campaigns on the role of diet and lifestyle prostate cancer. They might be successful in reaching men after they're diagnosed, but my goal was to reach men BEFORE symptoms—way before.

Also, they weren't engaged in campaigns to educate men living with prostate cancer on lifestyle interventions to improve outcomes. These issues weren't being addressed by the nonprofit he was heading or other nonprofit organizations. I told him this shouldn't be looked at as competition, but rather as another necessary voice to reach more men.

I set up a one-page website for Blue Cure that included my story, Blue Cure's mission and vision, a button to order Blue Cure T-shirts to raise start-up funds for the organization, and a Facebook button, which is where I wanted to drive users to connect and engage. The T-shirts had a big Blue Cure logo on the front and a phrase on the back that read, "Prostate Cancer: Not Just An Old Man's Disease." (I was the example that it wasn't an "old man's disease," though the data showed the opposite.)

In my mind, everyone who purchased these T-shirts was a walking billboard. I wanted people to ask them, "What is Blue Cure?" I felt encouraged when I received the first T-shirt order. And soon, more orders were received, and I read messages from prostate cancer survivors, wives, and children, thanking me for sharing my story and getting the word out about a disease they felt had low awareness. Some nights after I got home from work or an evening client event, I would fill fifteen or twenty T-shirt orders and write personal thank you notes I inserted in each package.

On November 16, 2010, I received a certificate of filing by the State of Texas for the Blue Cure Foundation, and on June 14, 2011, I received our 501(c)(3) nonprofit status from the IRS. That's when a Donate button was added to the one-page site, and our first goal was to raise funds to build an interactive website.

Blue Cure was official!

A few weeks after my diagnosis, I shared the news with my friend Sofia van der Dys, a commercial photographer I worked with on ad campaigns for clients. I wasn't sure how my diagnosis would affect my business and client relations, but I was anxious, and I vented my concerns to Sofia. I feared some of my clients would think I wasn't able to give them my full attention. (I understand the fear many men have in not sharing their diagnosis, especially men in positions of power.) Sofia was an encouraging voice and asked me to focus on my mental health and doctor's visits and not my fears about what my clients might say or do.

Sofia's husband is close to my age, and she has a son. Being diagnosed with prostate cancer at thirty-five caught her attention, especially what I was learning and sharing about diet and lifestyle. She kept up with what I posted on Facebook, and she agreed that prostate cancer and men's health issues weren't getting enough attention. I shared with Sofia that I wanted to do something about this, create a movement moving the needle on the disparity men's health issues receive, particularly prostate cancer and lifestyle. Knowing my background in media, marketing, and public relations, she was highly encouraging, "If anyone can do it, you can."

I updated Sofia when I was close to announcing Blue Cure. She offered to help in any way that she could. There was one person she asked me to meet that could be the catalyst to help Blue Cure get off the ground, her good friend Carolyn Farb.

Carolyn Farb is the acclaimed First Lady of Philanthropy in Texas. I knew of Carolyn, but we had never met. I grew up in Houston, always seeing her in the news and on newspaper and magazine covers. Her philanthropy is legendary, and when Carolyn called attention to a cause, her advocacy raised awareness that translated to hundreds of millions of funds raised for numerous organizations.

Sofia scheduled a lunch for the three of us, and before we all met, she asked me to read Carolyn's book, *The Fine Art of Fundraising*. I did.

I met Sofia and Carolyn for lunch. When Carolyn arrived, it was like a scene out of a movie. As she walked through the dining room, patrons turned around in their chairs, nodding and saying hello as she passed. Carolyn had a larger-than-life presence that captured everyone's attention. She commanded respect for her philanthropy.

Carolyn and Sofia spoke for a bit. Then Carolyn turned her attention to me and asked me to share my story and how I wanted to impact lives. I shared my experiences, what I was learning, and how and why that could benefit millions of men of all ages. I spoke from the heart about what was lacking and how adding my voice could immediately move men to act.

I didn't ask Carolyn for anything. She listened, she processed what I was telling her about diet, lifestyle, and cancer, she nodded in agreement at times, but she didn't say much. I couldn't read her body language. Carolyn took some notes as our lunch was winding down. She asked me to get her three or four Blue Cure T-shirts for a few of her friends. I didn't know what would come of our lunch.

That night, I received an email from Carolyn graciously thanking me again for lunch and for sharing my story and vision for Blue Cure. As I continued to scroll down on the email, there was a to-do list of action items that required my immediate attention.

I needed to follow up and schedule a date for a meeting with John Mendelsohn, MD, the president of MD Anderson Cancer Center. The next action item was for me to meet with the director of public relations at the luxury department store Neiman Marcus. Carolyn wrote they would host a launch event for Blue Cure that would include a Men's Fall Fashion show. She was also going to make an introduction to Dr. Rod Paige, the former United States secretary of education (2001–2005), himself a prostate cancer survivor. Carolyn ended the email by reminding me to bring her a few Blue Cure T-shirts. These were going to be sent to her friends Fran Drescher, the star of the '90s sitcom, *The Nanny*, and Sir Roger Moore, a prostate cancer survivor who played British secret intelligence agent 007 James Bond in seven films. Carolyn had reached out to Fran and Roger and shared my story and mission for Blue Cure, and they agreed to take a photo wearing a Blue Cure T-shirt to show support for the cause.

Carolyn moved at lightning speed.

I was floored. After I read her email, I just sat there in my home office, leaned back in my chair, hands behind my head, with a big smile. After my diagnosis, smiles were hard to come by. Now I had something to smile about. This lady who I had just met did all that because of what I shared with her. I couldn't help but think, in her decades of philanthropy, working with hundreds of organizations and causes, that my story and my vision struck a chord. She recognized prostate cancer and men's health issues deserved more attention.

This would be the beginning of a decade working closely with Carolyn and learning the secrets to her success. Over the years, I've been asked by many how Carolyn makes magic. The "magic" attributed to Carolyn's involvement with a cause that I've learned by watching her is believing in a cause, putting in the man-hours, cultivating relationships, making the "ask," and being persistent. She does all of that. For decades, like many Houstonians who have seen Carolyn all over the media, I had no idea until I worked with her: how tirelessly she works the phones, personalizing literally thousands of emails, and building decades of goodwill so that when she calls on someone, they come through. She is one of the most brilliant, hard-working individuals I have met.

John Mendelsohn

John Mendelsohn, MD, was president of the University of Texas MD Anderson Cancer from 1996 to 2011. He died in 2019 at age eighty-two from glioblastoma, an aggressive form of brain cancer.

I met with Dr. Mendelsohn at his office at MD Anderson. This is the meeting Carolyn facilitated for me to share my vision for Blue Cure. I shared my frustrations in my short but seemingly long journey and emotional roller coaster with prostate cancer. At the time, I had met with five urologists at four institutions, including MD Anderson Cancer Center.

As he listened to me sharing my experiences, he shook his head in disbelief and said, "It was recommended you have surgery?" He couldn't believe one of the doctors had told me I should have surgery for localized, early-stage prostate cancer.

To my surprise, Dr. Mendelson didn't take issue when I told him one of my doctors encouraged me to change my diet and lifestyle to slow and possibly reverse the progression of my early-stage prostate cancer. In fact, he applauded it and highly encouraged me to read the book *Anticancer* by David Servan-Schreiber.

He also suggested I meet with Lorenzo Cohen, PhD, the director of Integrative Medicine at MD Anderson Cancer Center.

I had previously exchanged emails with Lorenzo, who also recommended I read *Anticancer*. Dr. Mendelsohn advocated the power of lifestyle interventions and integrative medicine. He commended Blue Cure's lifestyle focus and mission to reach younger males and encouraged me to keep sharing my story.

Months after our meeting, Dr. Mendelsohn and I would be interviewed separately for *The C Word* documentary about lifestyle and cancer prevention, produced by Academy Award winner Morgan Freeman and Academy Award nominee Meghan O'Hara.

Years later, at a screening for *The C Word*, I moderated a panel of experts, and Dr. Mendelsohn was one of the panelists. Full circle, the man who encouraged me to read *Anticancer* and who emphasized the importance of lifestyle interventions was on the stage I was moderating and in the same documentary.

Dr. Mendelsohn spent an hour with me that day in 2011, validating what I was learning about the power of lifestyle. The encouragement from a renowned, highly respected, and knowledgeable medical doctor and researcher, who led the number-one-rated cancer center in America, gave me more inspiration and motivation to stay the course and spread the message to men that LIFESTYLE MATTERS!

Chad Gonsoulin

A few weeks after I learned I had prostate cancer, I shared the news with my longtime friends Chad and his wife, Geni. I hadn't told any friends, as I was still trying to process my diagnosis. They shared words of encouragement and support, and over the coming months, Chad sincerely and repeatedly offered, "If there's anything you need, please let me know."

Chad and I are about the same age. He's an actively involved father of three. He has a son and a father about my dad's age. I shared what I was going through. I kept him apprised of my doctor's visits and what I was learning about the role of diet and lifestyle. He was genuinely interested. Like me, he wasn't aware of any prostate cancer and men's health campaigns. He agreed there was low awareness and acknowledged the lack of education on a holistic approach to men's health and the role nutrition and lifestyle have on prostate cancer.

When I shared the vision for Blue Cure, it piqued Chad's interest. He came over to the house one evening, and we discussed ways to reach men our age. He mentioned his young son and said it's also important to encourage healthy habits with our youth. Chad had planted a seed, and he asked for a bundle of Blue Cure T-shirts for some friends. "Trust me," he said.

A week later, Chad texted me a photo. It was star NFL Houston Texans quarterback Matt Schaub, wearing a Blue Cure T-shirt. I had no idea that Chad and Geni were personal friends with Matt and his wife, Laurie. Chad is a humble, modest guy. He isn't one to brag about relationships or his entrepreneurial business successes. He told me to post the photo of Matt Schaub on social media and let people know that NFL Houston Texans quarterback Matt Schaub supports Blue Cure and raising awareness of lifestyle and prostate cancer and men's health to encourage men to act. Chad also said posting Matt's photo would capture the attention of young men. And it did.

Matt Schaub would be the first of many endorsements from professional athletes that Chad would secure. And those endorsements would garner attention for Blue Cure, opening doors, gaining the interest of media and men of all ages, especially younger men. I was hearing from men who were checking out Blue Cure's content on social media after seeing Matt Schaub's photo.

The next time I saw Chad, he handed me an envelope with an unexpected donation for Blue Cure. He said again, "I want to help. Let's get the word out there and make an impact. This is an important message." I asked Chad to join Blue Cure's board of directors.

Chad's recruitment wasn't over with Matt Schaub. He introduced his friend, NFL Pro Bowl Houston Texans center Chris Myers, to Blue Cure. The first time I met Chris and his wife Jenny, Chris was wearing a Blue Cure T-shirt, representing us by dropping the ceremonial first puck at a professional hockey game. The massive NFL center was incredibly nice and engaging, asking a lot of questions about my journey and Blue Cure. Chris would soon join Blue Cure's board of directors, serving as an invaluable supporter using his platform to raise awareness of Blue Cure's lifestyle message. Chris was in television commercials for Blue Cure, participated in media interviews, emceed events, and recruited fellow professional athletes to support our cause and events. Having his involvement, and that of other professional athletes, helped chip away at the stigma in men talking about our health. (I embraced the involvement of "hyper-masculine" football players to reach a swath of men who needed to hear our lifestyle message.)

September 16, 2011 – National Prostate Cancer Awareness Month

Steve Mauldin remembered meeting me twelve years earlier at NBC-WFOR in Miami, where he was the vice president and general manager. He had introduced me to his news director, who offered me a job as a reporter-in-training when I got back from my graduate internship at CNN London.

Since our last visit in 1999, Steve had battled Stage IV cancer and was a survivor. Now he was the president and general manager of CBS 2 and KCAL 9 in Los Angeles.

Steve's son, Michael, a friend from college, was following my prostate cancer journey on Facebook. He told his father I would be out in Los Angeles for a TV interview on another network, and Mr. Mauldin had me speak with his news director, who booked me for a live segment.

I was grateful for the opportunity to share my story, and because it was so uniquely different from what viewers receive, I hoped it would move men to act. Los Angeles is the number two media market in America, and an interview reaches a lot of eyeballs. After I said goodbye to Mr. Mauldin on my way out of the building, I paused and thought how quickly time had passed since I last saw him in Miami. A decade had passed in the blink of an eye. I wondered where my life would be if I had pursued a career in journalism and taken the opportunity at CBS in Miami. I found myself now in a situation where I could take that passion I had for journalism and put it to use.

From KCAL, I drove to the NBC Los Angeles studios in Burbank and met anchor Lucy Noland, former anchor I knew from CBS Houston. She arranged a live six-minute interview with lead anchor Colleen Williams, a renowned award-winning journalist and interviewer. It was a conversational six-minute interview. The format and length allowed depth, not just a soundbite, and it benefitted viewers. When the interview ended, and as I walked off set, Colleen stopped me to ask a few more questions. She seemed genuinely interested and told me my story was unique, and she encouraged me to keep sharing it with men.

Colleen's parting words might have been what she usually tells guests, but her words were more motivational fuel. I just had live, on-camera interviews at two top-rated stations in the number two media market with large viewership, and I had shared an important message with viewers. I was proud of myself. The Los Angeles trip gave me the confidence I needed to feel more comfortable doing more television interviews and speaking engagements.

Before I left Los Angeles for Houston, Lucy Noland called from NBC LA telling me she was interested in interviewing me for a story that would air at different times. This was a big opportunity. I moved back my departure to Houston a few days and scheduled the interview the next day with Lucy.

Coincidentally, that evening, I received a phone call from an executive at a prostate cancer nonprofit based in the Los Angeles area, letting me know he saw my interview with Colleen on NBC. He questioned why I hadn't informed him ahead of time I would be out in Los Angeles doing media. I didn't know what to make of the call. Why would I need to let him know I was in Los Angeles? The call and questioning were strange.

The next day, when I was back at NBC LA studios waiting to be interviewed, I looked at the computer screen next to where I was sitting and saw the prostate cancer nonprofit had ads running on the station's website. I wondered how large their ad buy was. I wondered if they also had television commercials airing. I wondered if they had received any media interviews with the station. It was National Prostate Cancer Awareness Month. I also wondered if their media buyer made calls and complained. I knew how it worked behind the scenes. Media, marketing, and public relations were my business and background. Sales and news divisions are separate, but many times I had placed media buys for clients, and I was able to secure news/editorial coverage. I got paranoid, thinking the interview I was about to tape would not air; however, I realized my small nonprofit was not a threat to any other organization.

I taped my interview with Lucy. It was a solid substantive interview. After, Lucy had me go with a three-person (producer, cameraman, lighting guy) crew to a park, where they taped me running sprints, performing push-ups and chin-ups. They needed the B-roll to run with my soundbites talking about my change in lifestyle habits. We were at the park for a few hours. I thought to myself, "No way this story won't air. Not with the time and resources they've put into this news package."

The story didn't air.

I checked online a few days later. Nothing.

Back in Houston, I called Lucy a week later and asked if the story would air. There was a long pause. She told me she didn't know. She didn't offer anything more. I didn't ask. I thanked her again for the opportunity to share my story. I checked online the rest of the month, and the following month. It never aired.

I had my suspicions.

Blue Cure's mission—the reason I started it—was not the focus of other prostate cancer nonprofit organizations. In 2010, when I was diagnosed, and in 2011, when I started Blue Cure, I was determined to change the way prostate cancer was covered by the media and to introduce the message of lifestyle interventions. I wanted to reach younger guys and help end the stigma men have in discussing our health issues. Planting seeds with younger men was necessary, and that was my hope in sharing my story.

Months later, I received a public comment on Blue Cure's Facebook page by a board member of another prostate cancer nonprofit. It was personal, attacking my character, calling me attention-seeking and selfish for not supporting their organization. I couldn't believe it. I was shocked, and I was hurt. Later that day, the president of that nonprofit organization called and apologized on behalf of the organization but also weirdly added, "I wish we had Fran Drescher and other celebrities wearing a T-shirt with our logo." I shook my head in disbelief. They were an established nonprofit organization, funded by major pharmaceutical companies, a staff, and a marketing and public relations team, and this was petty.

I had never heard of that nonprofit or any prostate cancer nonprofit before my diagnosis, until I began searching online for help and support. I didn't want Blue Cure to become known once someone had prostate cancer. I wanted men to know the message before their diagnosis. I wanted to help other men avoid an unexpected diagnosis and have knowledge about lifestyle and treatment options. I wanted Blue Cure to be the catalyst that had men schedule an annual checkup and an appointment with his urologist, to adopt healthier habits, and be open about discussing with others their mental and physical health.

Red Meat, Dairy, and Discomfort

It was September's National Prostate Cancer Awareness Month. Fox News Network had contacted me about a media interview. The producer learned from Philippa Cheetham, MD, a urologist who worked with Dr. Katz at Columbia University Medical, that I had been diagnosed at thirty-five, and because of my diagnosis at a younger age, it would be newsworthy to share my story. I wasn't in New York City and couldn't participate in an in-studio interview, but fortunately, I was interviewed, and my story was posted on FoxNews.com and disseminated on social media. The lifestyle changes recommended by my doctor were central to the piece, and that was important to be in the story. I received so much feedback from this piece as a result of Fox's massive reach.

Excerpt from the FoxNews.com article, "Prostate Cancer: Not Just an Old Man's Cancer":

> "Canales decided to change his lifestyle...he started eating organically and modified his diet. He cut out red meat and increased the amount of vegetables he ate.
>
> Dr. Philipa Cheetham, a board-certified urologist who specializes in prostate cancer at Columbia University Medical Center, said Canales may be onto something.
>
> 'There is an overwhelming amount of evidence to support diet and prostate cancer to both prostate cancer-causing foods and prostate cancer-protective foods,' she said. 'There is certainly evidence from more than twenty-five studies that support the fact that the more red meat a man eats, the higher his risk of developing the disease. There are also numerous studies that show fried foods, processed foods, saturated animal fats and a diet high in animal dairy increases the risk of prostate cancer – and can accelerate the progression of the disease in those who have it.'"[37]

I received a lot of questions from that article, and most of them were asking about Dr. Cheetham's statement about red meat and dairy. That was controversial for my Texas red meat-eating buddies who had never heard of a connection with diet and health, particularly between red meat and prostate cancer. I didn't make the statement; a medical doctor did. A lot of friends, family, and strangers found it hard to believe. I turned around and asked them if their doctors had ever given them any advice on healthy foods to prevent chronic disease and cancer. Everyone answered, "No." The active holistic surveillance protocol I was on called for me to not eat red meat, processed meat, no dairy products (no milk and cheese), no fried foods, no sugary drinks, and no sweets.

Up until the day I met Dr. Katz, I ate red and processed meats, drank milk, and consumed cheese. I understood the pushback from my friends. I wasn't finger-pointing and finger-wagging, telling them how to eat. I shared my story and what the doctors told me. Importantly, I shared what foods I was adding: lots of cruciferous vegetables, leafy green vegetables, legumes, nuts, seeds, and wild salmon (though today I eat a 100 percent whole-foods plant-based diet.)

Blue Cure Launch Event

The date had arrived for the Blue Cure-Neiman Marcus Men's Fall Fashion event at the Houston Galleria. This was promoted as Blue Cure's launch party. The Neiman Marcus team oversaw the event, and I had nothing to do with the planning and details. I was told to show up. The Neiman Marcus PR team did not disappoint. They went all out. In the entry to the store that faced heavy street traffic, there was a highly visible main window display that featured mannequins dressed in Blue Cure T-shirts, with a large Blue Cure logo hanging in the background. When you entered Neiman Marcus, you saw the display. When you drove by Neiman Marcus, you saw the display and that big Blue Cure logo. Each time I drove by Neiman Marcus and saw the display, I would tell myself, "There are people you don't know asking, 'What is Blue Cure?'" Some of these people will Google our website and learn about Blue Cure's mission and learn my story. Some will tell their dad; some will talk to their grandfather and their son. Some will schedule a doctor's visit and ask if they should get screened for prostate cancer.

I arrived at Neiman Marcus an hour before the event and saw they had built a runway for the fashion show with a large Blue Cure logo as the backdrop. Life-sized mannequins dressed in Blue Cure tees were placed all around the event, as were information cards sharing a summary of my story and Blue Cure's mission.

I didn't have expectations for the event. To my surprise, there were over three hundred attendees. There were quite a few faces of Houston influencers and business leaders that I recognized. Everyone was dressed like they were out of a fashion magazine. It was like a GQ event. I thought of my publicist friend in New York who told me about the men's fashion brand they proposed to do a blue campaign for men's health. She told me fashion presented a lot of opportunities for Blue Cure and myself.

I shook a lot of hands, thanked each person for attending and allowing me to share my story and my hopes for Blue Cure. I noticed there were a lot of female attendees. At least 80 to 90 percent of the attendees were women, and a lot of them were telling me the same thing, "There's not enough being done for men. There's not any attention on men's health and prostate cancer." Some of the women told me about their fathers and grandfathers who had been treated for prostate cancer. All of them were surprised to learn I wasn't having surgery or radiation and instead was "treating" my early-stage prostate cancer with dietary and lifestyle interventions. They had never heard of that, and I saw the look of surprise. Many of the women told me the men in their life didn't like talking about their health. I understood. There was a stigma. Most of the men I spoke with listened and didn't ask questions.

The men's fashion show got underway, and the male models walked the runway dressed in the latest fall fashion. At the end of the show, they all walked out clapping, wearing Blue Cure T-shirts. The Neiman Marcus PR director handed me the microphone and asked me to stand in the middle of the runway and address the three-hundred-plus attendees who had come to support Blue Cure. I wasn't prepared to give a speech, and to say I was nervous is an understatement. As a marketing and public relations strategist, I am aware of how moments can be perceived. Control was part of my personality, and not preparing a speech and being asked to address a large crowd resulted in my anxiety shooting up.

My palms were sweating. I looked down as I walked to the center of the runway, cleared my throat, and mumbled some words. I paused, took a deep breath, looked up, and saw the hundreds of faces staring at me. I told myself, "C'mon, Gabe! They came to support you and learn about Blue Cure."

I locked eyes with a few people in the front row and spoke to them so I would tune out all the faces staring at me. My words were brief, expressing my gratitude. I thanked everyone for coming to support Blue Cure, and I encouraged the mostly female attendees to get the men in their lives to get a checkup and discuss screenings with their doctor.

I received a lot of positive feedback and interest after the event, but for days, I dwelled on those last few moments when I didn't feel I was at my best. I didn't like that I could have been perceived as lacking confidence when I spoke. I also didn't like that I had to focus on a few faces in the front row to share my gratitude. I wanted to look around at everyone that was there, look into their eyes and give thanks. My controlling nature had me focus on what I perceived as the bad part of the event and not the good that came from it. What's crazy is I was so worried about what others were thinking when they probably weren't giving my short speech a second thought.

An emphasis of Dr. Katz's active holistic surveillance protocol was for me to manage stress. Dr. Servan-Schreiber wrote about the importance of stress management in *Anticancer*. It was key to the *Anticancer* lifestyle. Dr. Lorenzo Cohen also emphasized it. I was getting the message on different fronts: I had to confront my anxiety issues and focus on my mental health. I was working on it. It would be a process. Like my dietary habits, my mental health strategies would be the key to transforming my lifestyle habits. They would go together.

Celebrity

The power of celebrity is undeniable. Like professional athletes, celebrities from television, film, and music are very influential and have legions of passionate followers. Carolyn getting Fran Drescher and Roger Moore to take photos wearing Blue Cure T-shirts played a role in me securing media interviews. It added to the intrigue when discussing Blue Cure and the issues I was raising. When I was interviewed on television in Houston, New York, Los Angeles, Portland, and Seattle, photos of Fran and Roger wearing Blue Cure T-shirts would be shown during the segment.

Both Fran and Roger were cancer survivors—Fran, a uterine cancer survivor, and Roger, a prostate cancer survivor. Roger passed away from liver cancer in 2017. Unfortunately, I didn't get the chance to meet him and his wife, Lady Kristina, and personally thank them for their support.

Fran Drescher is the actress who played the iconic Fran Fine in the '90s hit television series, *The Nanny*. Fran wrote the 2002 *New York Times* bestselling book *Cancer Schmancer*, detailing her journey with cancer. Fran is the founder of Cancer Schmancer, which is "dedicated to educating, motivating, and activating patients into medical consumers by connecting lifestyle to disease."[38]

I corresponded with Fran via email and thanked her for publicly supporting Blue Cure, and I was able to personally thank her when we met at a Cancer Schmancer benefit at the Pasadena Playhouse on September 25, 2012, in California. She was as nice as I had imagined.

Fran spoke after the benefit performance and took questions. I sat in the front, watching how passionately she spoke about her cancer journey, cancer prevention, environmental factors, and what it means to be a proactive medical consumer. She had command of what she was talking about, she believed in what she was saying, and she was passionate about the "why." She was authentic and vulnerable, and that resonated with me and, I'm sure, with everyone in the auditorium. I was captivated. She had command and passion about what she shared. I looked around, and everyone was nodding as she spoke. I was moved to act and do more, but at the same time, I found myself intimidated. I realized I didn't know a fraction of what Fran was talking about. Was I ready to be doing what I was doing with Blue Cure? Doubt reared its ugly head. I spent some time talking to Fran when the Q&A ended to let her know how inspired I was and thanked her for her cancer advocacy. There is value in learning from the experiences of others.

That night when I got back to my hotel room, two things came over me. I realized the intimidation I felt about what I didn't know was a good thing, because I don't know everything. I'm on a journey to learn as much as I can every day. So, I used that feeling of insecurity to encourage myself that there's more to learn, to not feel shame and intimidation about what I don't know. The other realization about that evening was the way Fran spoke connected with people. It was because she was authentic and vulnerable. She shared knowledge and how she felt. I realized for me to have a greater impact with men and families, it would be important for me to be more vulnerable and to share how I had felt during my journey, and when I share the stories of others, to include those elements. Authenticity is powerful.

Fran Drescher and the Cancer Schmancer organization shared content from Blue Cure's social media to their hundreds of thousands of fans and supporters, including my 2013 TED talk, which would take place a year later.

America is a celebrity-driven culture. When celebrities spotlight a cause, it moves others to act. I've been fortunate and grateful when celebrities spotlight Blue Cure. It's opened the minds of men to learn about lifestyle and men's health and the connection with cancer and disease.

Many celebrities would lend their support in a petition I initiated in 2014 to light the White House blue.

Sharing in a Position of Power

Dr. Rod Paige served as the seventh United States secretary of education from 2001 to 2005. He's the first African American to serve in that role, and, a little history, he was with President George W. Bush at the Emma E. Booker Elementary School in Sarasota, Florida when the president received news that a second plane had hit the World Trade Center on September 11, 2001.

Dr. Paige is also a prostate cancer survivor. You may not recall reading or hearing about it, because it wasn't in the news. Shortly after the Neiman Marcus launch event, Carolyn Farb scheduled a lunch for the three of us. Carolyn and Rod were close longtime friends. I shared my story, family history of chronic disease, and reason for starting Blue Cure, and Dr. Paige shared a little about his cancer journey.

Carolyn told Dr. Paige why she was supporting Blue Cure and directly asked Dr. Paige for his public support. Without hesitation, he agreed to support Blue Cure. That's how much weight Carolyn Farb's endorsement carried. Carolyn brought a Blue Cure T-shirt for Dr. Paige and asked if he could put it on for a photo that would be posted on social media. Dr. Paige agreed, excused himself to go to the men's room, and a few minutes later was wearing a Blue Cure T-shirt with his suit pants, and the three of us took photos.

That photo was important for me to publicly share on Facebook since Dr. Paige is an African American survivor of prostate cancer. I had learned of the racial disparities of African American men and prostate cancer incidence and death. I knew the African American community, like the Hispanic community and my Hispanic family, had higher rates of chronic diseases. They were more overweight and suffered from obesity. There needed to be more attention on these disparities and more encouragement for African American and Hispanic men to get annual checkups and adopt healthy lifestyle habits.

A few months after that lunch, Dr. Paige and I met for breakfast. Gone was the formality of the first meeting. Dr. Paige and I met in workout clothes, and perhaps because it was just the two of us, two men, Dr. Paige felt more comfortable sharing more details about his experience with prostate cancer. His cancer had been a lot more aggressive than he shared in our previous lunch. As a Hispanic man, I had seen up close the effects of "machismo" cultural norms with men in my family who died prematurely due to unhealthy habits and not scheduling annual checkups. Awareness and education were sorely needed among Hispanic and African American men. Representation mattered, and I wanted to use my story, and Dr. Paige's story, to purposefully target Hispanics and African Americans with the message of lifestyle and prevention and encourage routine checkups.

Dr. Paige would join Blue Cure's board of directors, and in 2013, he would be the honoree at Blue Cure's Inaugural Lecture Series.

A Journalist's Belief

In early 2012, I met journalist Lily Jang. She had just moved back home to Houston from Seattle, where she had been a longtime news anchor at Q13 FOX. Lily was the new morning anchor for KHOU, the Houston CBS affiliate.

I was at a coffee bar when I happened to read an article about Lily moving back to Houston. Just as I lifted my eyes from reading that article, Lily stood a few feet away. What a coincidence! I went over and introduced myself, welcoming her back to her hometown.

Lily was engaging, conversational, asking what I did and if I enjoyed it. I told her I owned a marketing company but was devoting more and more of my energy to Blue Cure. I shared why I started it. She seemed genuinely surprised when I shared that I was living with prostate cancer, and she was interested in learning more about my story. Lily told me a little about her father having health issues, which was a big reason for her move back to Houston. She agreed that prostate cancer and men's health issues needed more attention. Lily was on her way to a meeting but wanted to continue the conversation.

She reached out to me a few weeks later, letting me know she wanted to support Blue Cure and share my story. I was grateful and thought we were about to schedule a television interview. That wasn't it. She wanted Blue Cure to be the beneficiary for a CBS-KHOU-sponsored event that would include heavy promotion and media coverage. It would take place at Hotel ZaZa, a popular swanky hotel in Houston's Museum District. I jumped at the opportunity, and I knew it would give Blue Cure a huge boost in name recognition.

The event was called "Tweetup for Blue Cure" and was scheduled during June for Men's Health Month. It was a first of its kind for a news station in Houston (and, as far as I know, the first of its kind in America), harnessing the reach of Twitter and social media influencers to educate Houstonians on issues surrounding prostate cancer. KHOU ran a lot of commercials promoting the event, and Lily interviewed me for news segments. I was able to share my prostate cancer journey, raise awareness of the connection between lifestyle and prostate cancer, and highlight the importance of men having a conversation with their doctor about getting screened.

Forty-plus valet, hotel, and event staff wearing Blue Cure T-shirts and blue Converse sneakers greeted the more than five hundred attendees. The blue-themed event Hotel ZaZa's team created was high-energy, with Gaudi-esque blue decor, and blue lasers. A DJ played music outside next to a dance floor that had been constructed that morning with string lights overhead. Inside was a live band. The crowd was shoulder to shoulder, many dancing, others socializing. Big screens hung outside displaying live tweets about prostate cancer with a group of urologists and healthcare professionals on hand to answer and reply to live tweets. There were journalists and media personalities from various outlets, players from the NFL Houston Texans, high-profile business leaders, government officials and community influencers, and KHOU viewers who showed up to support it.

It was over-the-top fun. I shook hundreds of hands. It was challenging to have a conversation, but I made new friends that would be long-lasting in support of Blue Cure. The "Tweetup for Blue Cure" was covered by the local papers and monthly magazines. Quite a few attendees went out of their way to let me know they had never been to an event in support of men's health and prostate cancer. I wasn't surprised. My hope was the media and promotion that surrounded the event would lead to more attention to men's health issues and would encourage men to visit the doctor.

Over the next three years, Hotel ZaZa and KHOU hosted these highly promoted and publicized Blue Cure events, which raised a lot of awareness of lifestyle and prostate cancer. Hotel ZaZa also sponsored one large Blue Cure for Prostate Cancer event in Dallas. I was grateful and fortunate to have these opportunities to share an important message. I received lots of positive feedback and questions. I heard from men who were inspired to get a checkup, get a PSA, and eat healthier.

CHAPTER TWELVE

HYPOCRISY

As the years went by, I worried about whether Blue Cure's lifestyle message was clouded by these parties. For good reason. I started believing there was a disconnect with myself. I didn't want to be perceived as a hypocrite.

Every day, I looked for articles and research on the role of diet and lifestyle on prostate cancer and chronic disease. It was my interest, and it was my job to become educated and informed. As I gained knowledge, my habits changed. It wasn't easy. Sometimes it was two steps forward, one step back, and there were periods when it was one step forward, two steps back. My environment was essential to my daily success or possible long-term setback.

I had been going to therapy for a few years to deal with my anxiety and bouts of depression, and I had gained awareness of my triggers and how to pivot when they arose. After my diagnosis, I stopped drinking. I just quit cold turkey. I needed to because of the ripple effect it had on other lifestyle habits.

The first event at Hotel ZaZa, the Tweetup for Blue Cure, was a setback for me personally. That evening was the first I had a drink since my diagnosis. My doctor had encouraged me not to drink.

I'm not blaming anyone for my actions. It's on me. I was talking to hundreds of people, and everyone had a drink in hand. Servers passed by every few minutes offering hors d'oeuvres, drinks, and shots. I was anxious. One person after another asked, "Why aren't you having a drink?" The professional athletes were drinking; the doctors were drinking. The pull was too strong. I chose to "be social" and have a drink, but then I had another, and another, one more. It was me, pre-diagnosis, when I would down vodka-sodas very quickly so I would feel more relaxed, able to more easily engage in conversation. There was a lot of drinking that evening. A few friends had to get rides home because they were drunk, the responsible thing to do, but not what I expected. No one said anything to me about my drinking. That night, after the party and on the way home, I stopped at a fast food drive-through, double-ordered fried chicken strips and cream gravy, large fries, a and large Coke.

The next day, I was physically exhausted. I was dehydrated and dealt with a pounding headache that lasted all day. I felt like shit. I was mad at myself for how my drinking throughout the night could be perceived. I wasn't finger-wagging, telling people not to drink, but binge drinking wasn't the message I wanted to portray.

Drinking that evening was a trigger that set me back to occasionally having a drink at dinner or at an event. Sometimes one drink became two or three, four, five, or six. I would make an excuse to myself that it was occasionally, it was "in moderation," but then I would eat bar food and unhealthy junk food I had proudly stayed away from since Dr. Katz's recommendation when I visited him in New York.

I hated that I would fall back into old habits, and I would continue to make excuses—"I'm not eating red meat like before," or "I'm not eating as much fried foods as before." A trigger would have a ripple effect and could quickly lead to a huge crashing wave of weight gain, guilt, and shame.

I wrestled with whether we should put a pause on the big parties. I recognize there's a tremendous opportunity to plant seeds of change in environments that aren't health settings. On the other hand, I looked at the amount of time and resources that had been put into each event and considered putting just as much energy promoting an event that was 100 percent focused on promoting a healthy lifestyle, with all activities, food, and beverages mirroring the healthy, anti-cancer message I was advocating.

Carmel-By-The-Sea

After spending a transformative week recharging in Carmel-by-the-Sea, California, breathing in fresh air, spending time in nature, hiking (sometimes as much as eight to ten miles a day), I enjoyed the fresh fruits and vegetables grown in the nearby Salinas Valley and walking around town. I was inspired to make more lifestyle changes.

That visit to the West Coast had such a profound impact on me. I thought of how I could "bring Carmel back to Houston." When I got back to Houston, it wasn't long before (one day) I recognized my anxiety increased as I navigated the Houston traffic in my hour commute from my suburban home to the office. I was always on a call when I was on the road. When the traffic slowed to a crawl, I checked emails on my phone. I was too connected, morning and night, and I knew it wasn't healthy.

I decided the week I got back from Carmel that I needed to move from my house in the suburbs to a place close to the office, within walking distance, close to a gym and grocery store. My lease on my SUV was up, and I had been looking at new cars. I decided that once I made the move into town, close to the office, I would not get another car. I decided to purchase a bike. That way, I wouldn't always be on the phone or texting and returning emails while stuck in traffic. When I needed to attend a meeting that required me to wear a suit, I would take an Uber.

And that's what I did. I didn't know how long it would last (six years). I made those changes and didn't regret it for one second. I had to. Stress management was key in reversing the progression of my early-stage prostate cancer. It also saved me hours of commute time on the road, allowed me to disconnect from my phone, and discover many new places around town. I increased my movement, walked around more, and explored the numerous parks and bike paths in Houston. I couldn't move to Carmel-by-the-Sea, but I looked at what I could do to create less stress for myself back in Houston.

Those lifestyle changes inspired me in numerous ways. I asked CBS-KHOU if they would support and sponsor a prostate cancer run that would promote healthy lifestyle habits. KHOU said yes, and Lily Jang agreed to serve as the emcee. I knew creating an event like this would help me personally and serve as a better vehicle to promote Blue Cure's anti-cancer lifestyle message.

My initial idea to promote the lifestyle message at the Blue Cure Run was to partner with a farmer's market to promote the benefits of eating more plants. I wanted our run to have local and regional farmers selling their produce, vendors providing samples of healthy foods, smoothies, and cooking demonstrations. I also envisioned having a yoga session before the event to promote the practice and encourage stretching and mindfulness. I started planning the event, meeting with city officials, and in the meantime, another event that I was asked to be a part of would influence the direction of the Blue Cure Run.

Ride of a Lifetime

In 2014, representatives from the MD Anderson Cancer Center asked me to emcee the Ride of a Lifetime event to promote cancer prevention. This was the first event I was aware of hosted by a major cancer center that solely promoted cancer prevention through exercise and a healthy lifestyle. I couldn't wait to see how MD Anderson produced the event and what kind of response it would receive.

Ride of a Lifetime was an outdoor two-hour cycling class followed by one hour of Zumba, which I understood to be a Latin-inspired cardio dance workout. My mother took a Zumba class with her friends, but I had never seen it and didn't know what to expect. I was in for a surprise.

Three hundred stationary cycling bikes were stationed in an outdoor courtyard of a popular city center in Houston. Large flat-screen televisions were set on high pedestals placed throughout the event area, displaying key messages for cancer prevention. A large stage for the cycling leaders was front and center of the cyclists, and a high-rise building served as a backdrop. There was an information booth with educational brochures on cancer prevention and plenty of staff and volunteers from MD Anderson Cancer Center. There was an MD Anderson Cancer Center "End Cancer" display to sign with a message for yourself or a loved one who has faced cancer.

After I welcomed participants, I introduced cancer survivors who took to the stage and shared their cancer journeys. There were tears and cheers, and you couldn't help but be inspired by the stories shared. I was choked up.

Music filled the air. I felt the stage vibrate from the bass as I exited. The cycling instructor took over getting the crowd pumped up, and they responded with a loud roar. They were ready to cycle for cancer prevention.

When the cycling class ended, there was a thirty-minute transition when the production team and army of staffers quickly removed the bikes.

It was now dark, and hundreds gathered in front of the lit stage ready to Zumba. The hundreds turned to over a thousand. Lasers beamed over the heads of the gathered, and laser art and light projections illuminated the surrounding buildings. The music started, the Zumba instructor took the stage, and a sea of participants moved in unison. The lights, lasers, dance music, and mass of participants made for a concert-like atmosphere. The thousand-plus, mostly women, crowded the tight outdoor courtyard, including my mother, who brought a group of girlfriends. It was a sight to see women of all ages, in their teens, twenties, fifties through eighties, enthusiastically moving to the beats with so much energy, dripping in sweat, and playfully shouting at the instructor. Around five hundred onlookers packed the sides and danced. Zumba extended from a scripted one hour to almost two hours, and the participants didn't want it to end, with shouts of "No!" as the instructor said they had to wind down.

It was a high-energy event that made a big impression on me—so much so that I changed the Blue Cure Run to the Blue Cure Night Run and added Zumba to draw women, influencers of men, who might not want to run. Overall cancer prevention would be a big part of promoting the run.

I hired one of the production teams that worked on Ride of a Lifetime. I was ready to create a fun and informative experience for dads, sons, brothers, grandfathers, and the women who love them.

Blue Cure Night Run

A run seemed like a great idea, but I didn't consider hurricane season and Houston's unforgiving thunderstorms.

I scheduled the Blue Cure Night Run (BCNR) during September's National Prostate Cancer Awareness Month. There was already a morning prostate cancer run that took place months earlier around Father's Day in downtown Houston, but prostate cancer and men's health issues had such low awareness and media attention. I believed a second run three and a half months apart was not an issue. The Blue Cure Night Run would have a strong emphasis on diet, lifestyle, and prostate cancer, and it would encourage all men to schedule an annual checkup.

I was able to secure a park on the western edge of downtown Houston, with the historic City Hall illuminated blue and the downtown skyline as a picturesque backdrop. The mayor's office agreed to our request to light City Hall blue the evening of our event.

In the planning stages of the event, I met with a Houston city official who oversaw permitting. He told me to manage my expectations about turnout and said there was a decrease in participation in most of the Houston runs due to saturation of run events. Too many runs had been permitted, and multiple runs were scheduled every Saturday and each weekend of the year. The city official told me even the popular runs had recently experienced a severe decrease in registrations. I wasn't deterred.

I recognized that a lot of nonprofits and organizations were scheduling runs, and for us to stand out and get our message out, we had to be different. The 2014 Blue Cure Night Run would be the first 5K event I would plan and be a part of. I had no frame of reference. I had never run in a 5K or a fun run, but I had attended many events and produced a few. So, in my mind, it was about creating an event that would be an experience for our participants. I wanted to replicate the energy I felt at Ride of a Lifetime. I wanted to create a memorable experience that would lead to Monday morning watercooler conversations. And most importantly, I wanted to plant seeds so participants would want to learn more about anti-cancer living. I wanted to cultivate a desire to adopt healthy lifestyle habits and schedule a checkup with a doctor. But whether we had one hundred participants or a thousand, for me, it was using the event as a vehicle to promote our message.

I hired a race director, who helped with the planning and management of the event. His advice was to keep it simple: participants would get a race

T-shirt, run or walk the route, grab a beer, and then go home. That wasn't my vision.

The city official told me registrations were on the decline, so we had to add different elements. It would be a nighttime event, which already made it different. We would have yoga and Zumba. Participants would receive a T-shirt, blue glow sticks, and necklaces. We would have a DJ and entertainment; vendors would offer plant-based snacks and healthy beverages. No alcoholic beverages would be offered, and we would have lasers and lights beaming on buildings and in the park. This would be a family-friendly event that would promote anti-cancer living and prostate cancer education.

The race director encouraged me to rethink not offering alcohol and said many runs provided a beer or two when runners finish. I was approached and offered sponsor dollars to partner with an alcoholic brand. I declined. I'm not finger-wagging or finger-pointing. I wanted our family-friendly event to spotlight food and lifestyle that promote good health and anti-cancer living, and alcohol wasn't in the mix. I got a lot of pushback from people involved who said we should offer it, but our medical advisory board members agreed we shouldn't have big beer banners and bottles of beer handed out at our event. I also recognized my challenges with alcohol and triggers, a challenge other family members and friends also experience. I was reminded that this was a fundraising event and that we needed funds to have education and advocacy programs to reach men, so I should be open to receiving sponsor dollars from alcohol breweries. I didn't budge. Our event didn't have any big-dollar sponsors from Big Pharma, Big Food, Big Soda—just a few local paying sponsors and in-kind sponsors. It was a challenge.

Three weeks out from the 2014 Blue Cure Night Run, our registrations were around a few hundred. The race director told me that with fun runs and 5Ks, registrations increase dramatically leading up to the event. Our number of registrations increased a few weeks out and exploded the week of the run, with onsite registration taking us over 1,000. It was gratifying to see a sea of blue with all the participants wearing their bright Blue Cure race tank tops. I met people of all ages, prostate cancer survivors, wives, and daughters running on behalf of a father who passed from prostate cancer.

Lots of younger families, and surprisingly, as I shook hands to thank supporters, most that I met were there to support men's health. They had no connection to prostate cancer, but they had a father, brother, or grandfather who had passed away from a heart attack or was living with diabetes. They were there to support the men in their lives.

The 5K run was complete. Participants visited our vendor tents, getting plant-based snacks, and our emcee was getting the crowd ready for Zumba. I worried the runners would just head home after the run, but many stuck around to watch Zumba, and when they saw the fun and felt the Zumba energy, many joined in, including men. There was a large group of women who had registered for the Blue Cure Night Run only to participate in Zumba. Some had printed or painted on their shirts "For my husband" and "For my dad."

As the event ended, every person that passed me on their way back to their car gave me a high-five or a nod, letting me know it was a great event and they would be back. Female attendees provided most of the positive feedback, with many commenting on the need for more events "for our men."

After the inaugural 2014 Night Run, Blue Cure hosted run events in 2015 and 2016. The 2017 event was rescheduled due to Hurricane Harvey. But we hosted two in 2018 and one in 2019. The 2020 one was canceled due to the pandemic, but we finished 2021 with a successful run in November. Our media partners CBS KHOU 11 and 104.1 KRBE were instrumental in getting our message out to hundreds of thousands of Houstonians. Having supportive station management and top broadcasting talents like Lily Jang and Ryan Chase serving as our emcees and using their social media and broadcasting platforms to promote our runs and educate the community helped us reach many in the community that benefitted from a prompting. Media partners and coverage make a huge difference in making an impact. I've met men years later who said they had seen a promo spot for our run or listened to a radio interview, and though they didn't attend the run, it pushed them to schedule a checkup, and that made a difference.

CHAPTER THIRTEEN

THE POWER OF GETTING SOCIAL

May 2012

I was doing my daily morning news search on Google and social media on "prostate cancer," "men's health," and "cancer" when I came across a *Forbes* headline, "How Facebook Is Changing the World for Good." I clicked on the link. Writer Rahim Kanani interviewed Libby Leffler, the strategic partner manager at Facebook. To my surprise, I was mentioned in the article.

> "Take Gabe Canales for example. In the winter of 2010, at the age of 35, Gabe was diagnosed with prostate cancer, and he felt overwhelmed with questions. After posting the details of his diagnosis on his Facebook profile, Gabe saw a flood of responses from friends, family and supporters, including questions from people who were going through the same thing, either personally or with a family member. So, Gabe decided to launch a Facebook Page called "Journey with Prostate Cancer". The Page quickly grew to a community of more than 7,000 people, becoming a crucial support and education network for Gabe, his friends and family, and others who are fighting a similar battle. Using Facebook, Gabe created a place for people to connect, share their experiences, and engage in authentic

and open dialogue about important issues. This is one of many examples in which people are using Facebook to reach out to friends and broader communities to address some of the most challenging issues we face."

—Libby Leffler[39]

The Journey with Prostate Cancer Facebook page was my outlet to share my feelings, my experiences, what I was learning, and to post articles I felt would benefit others.

I didn't seek out, nor did I feel comfortable attending an in-person support group. I was seeing my therapist. She encouraged me to journal and share my feelings and fears with family and friends, and I slowly began to.

I searched, and I couldn't find Facebook pages for men with prostate cancer and information on nutrition, lifestyle, stress management, nor did I find pages where men with prostate cancer were posting and sharing their experiences with specific treatments. I was inundated with questions from friends and acquaintances about my diagnosis. I received many posts, comments, and private messages on my Facebook profile. I decided to start the Journey with Prostate Cancer Facebook page as an extension of my notebook journaling my therapist had given me as one of my mental health exercises. This Facebook page was my "bridge" to connect with others going through a similar journey.

When developing social media strategies for my business clients, I emphasized their social media content should educate, inform, and be authentic to develop a connection with their consumers and prospects. I believed content that repeatedly solicited and sold to an audience wasn't the best way to engage and develop a long-term customer. That's how I thought of my Journey with Prostate Cancer Facebook page. It needed to be authentic, encourage dialogue, and post content I learned from, because I believed others would too and find it had value.

After reading the *Forbes* piece, I contacted Libby at Facebook and thanked her for sharing a piece of my story and how I chose to use Facebook to foster authentic conversations with men and families going through their prostate cancer journey. She listened as I shared the mental health challenges I had experienced after my diagnosis, not feeling comfortable attending an in-person support group, and finding some comfort and connection when I engaged with others on the Journey with Prostate Cancer Facebook page. I told her that some of those connections led to in-person meetings, and I was encouraged to learn others had met through the Journey with Prostate Cancer page and met in person too. It was also their bridge to connect.

During our conversation, Libby invited me to Facebook's headquarters in Menlo Park, California. She asked if I would share my story, which would be broadcast live on the Facebook for Nonprofits page. Libby told me I was using the platform in a way that should be recognized and shared with other nonprofits and others who could benefit.

Getting that invitation was an acknowledgment of what I was doing and was a much-needed validation. At times, I doubted what I was doing. I wondered if I was wasting my time and energy, if I was actually helping others and making any kind of a difference.

I flew into San Francisco and drove down to Menlo Park. I wasn't sure what to expect as I drove onto the campus of the world's largest social media company. I think I expected some futuristic-looking set of buildings, but it turns out the Facebook campus looked like many other office parks. I checked in with security, and a few minutes later, Libby came out to greet me and took me on a tour. I immediately noticed lots of young faces. I felt like I was back at college. They were focused on their screens, typing away on their keyboards. Most looked younger than me, some looked around my age. I wondered if they knew anything about their prostates. Did they get checkups? Or were they like me, thinking health problems aren't a concern for young guys?

I followed Libby to the studio. I wrote about the experience in *The Huffington Post*:

> We discussed how I used Facebook to start the Blue Cure prostate cancer nonprofit. We also discussed my belief that Facebook offers something profound in our "War on Cancer," by connecting families and offering support like never before, while offering education on much-needed

preventative dietary and lifestyle habits and on an integrative approach to fighting cancer.

If other cancer institutions and nonprofits would place such emphasis on using this powerful interactive medium for education and support, we could make incredible advances in our "War on Cancer."

More than anything, I've found through Blue Cure's Facebook interactions that the #1 need of cancer patients and their caregivers on a cancer journey is this: hope.

Hope in a cure.

Hope that all will be well.

Hope for a life-extending treatment.

Hope that someone can comfort them.

Hope that someone can connect with them who can relate and offer encouragement.

Hope.

Facebook offers patients and caregivers hope by providing a way to instantly connect like never before in human history.

Instant connectivity and interactivity takes this very big world — this scary new cancer-world, for some of us — and lets us intimately connect, receive support, become educated and become empowered. Such instant connections are a way to know immediately about new treatments and clinical trials and to share experiences about drugs, doctors, hospitals, treatments and other elements of the cancer journey.

In this way, Facebook is an essential weapon in our arsenal for the "War on Cancer," a war where geography is no longer a boundary. It's a place where knowledge and experiences are shared, instant feedback is provided and strangers bond quickly as friends. As dominant media was in early decades, TV and radio never offered this. Facebook does.

The cancer community must embrace this interactive medium — not just as a fundraising tool, as most do, but to empower, offer support and educate. (Diet and lifestyle choices not only can reduce cancer risks and prevent cancer but enable better outcomes when undergoing cancer treatments.)[40]

Social media has evolved greatly since I wrote that piece in 2012, and we have seen it used in nefarious ways. But I still believe social media can serve as a bridge to help men connect and meet in person if they eventually desire, find resources, and learn.

For my mental health, I unfollow and unfriend accounts that disseminate lots of negative information. Keep in mind that how we spend our time and what we read, watch, and listen to affects our mental health. The Blue Cure Facebook page currently has 230,000 followers and continues to provide information on cancer and disease prevention, prostate cancer screenings and treatments, as well as issues that affect men's mental and physical health.

Ted Talks

On October 12, 2013, I gave a TED Talk in Houston. My talk was titled, "Changing the Way We Fight Cancer."[41]

I heard from a few individuals that they had nominated me to give a TED Talk. They read and watched interviews of me and told me I was sharing information and experiences about prostate cancer they had never heard before, especially from a guy my age, and I should share that with a TED Talk. By that point, I was three years into living with early-stage prostate cancer. I knew I had to do it. I needed that stage and the TED Talks platform to share my message, so I jumped at the opportunity. I went through a series of interviews, was selected, and told to prepare a talk no longer than eighteen minutes.

I had never given a speech longer than a few minutes. Fear set in. I thought about the impromptu speech I gave in front of hundreds at the Blue Cure launch event, another speech I gave in Oregon shortly after, and other talks when my anxiety shot through the roof. Interestingly, I didn't have the same anxiety attacks and fears when I had TV and radio interviews, but being in front of crowds was different. I assumed it was all in my preparation and that I needed to prepare differently to gain confidence and feel more comfortable. If I'm being honest with myself, I didn't feel "worthy" speaking in front of large groups.

I was committed and had to get my TED Talk right. I wanted my message to move audience members to act. Worrying I would look like a fool on stage, I started researching how to give persuasive talks, but eighteen minutes was daunting! I found a communications expert who had worked with well-known business leaders in developing powerful presentations. I contacted her office and inquired about a consultation. She was offering a workshop at her company headquarters in California, and I decided to make the trek.

I knew what I wanted to say but worried about how to say it and how it would be received. Of course, I had no control over what people would think, but I didn't want people to not be moved in some way from it. After going through the workshop, I gained more confidence. I wrote down my talk, began memorizing and rehearsing.

The morning of my TED Talk, I didn't feel good. I didn't sleep the night before, tossing and turning, that voice in my head telling me, "you're not worthy." I was worried it wouldn't be perfect and I would mess up. I was filled with negative thoughts of what could go wrong. That morning,

I threw up, the voice in my head telling me, "Cancel! Get out of it! Don't go! Save yourself the humiliation."

I arrived at Rice University, the site of that year's TEDx Houston. I went into the men's room, splashed water on my face, and stared in the mirror at those dark purplish, grey circles under my eyes and thought, "God, you look like hell." I did. I looked like I had been drinking all night. I hadn't.

I looked at my phone, which I had set on silent, and saw I had four missed calls from my mother. I called back, worried, thinking something was wrong, but she had called to wish me luck. She heard it in my voice, and she knew. I told her I hadn't slept; I wasn't going to do well. I threw up.... I was rambling negativity, and my mother interrupted and, with a raised voice, said, "You've lived this for almost three years. This is your story. This is your journey. Speak from the heart. Share what you've learned. Share what you've experienced and share why men need to hear it! DO NOT WORRY how it will be received. That's out of your hands!"

After the call, I just stood there and marinated on her words.

I stood to the side of the stage and heard the thunderous applause for the speaker before me, who had just finished. A few minutes went by, my name was called, and I walked to the center, telling myself, "This is your story. It's your journey. You can help others. Speak from the heart." I looked up and saw six hundred faces staring at me.

I started and went off-script from the outline I had memorized. The words began to flow, and I went into a zone. The fear was gone, no nerves. I just shared my journey and made a point. I finished and heard the applause. Obligatory applause? I wasn't sure. I was happy it was over, and I felt good about what I said.

After my talk, there was an intermission, and I made my way to the lobby to grab a water. I was met with a small crowd of attendees around me. They gave me positive feedback on my talk. They let me know that my talk gave them a lot to think about. They asked more questions about my experiences with doctors, prostate health, and my mental health. Someone showed me an impressive sketch he made during my talk of phrases and points I made that stood out to him. He told me he was going to throw out everything in his fridge when he got home and schedule a checkup. He was moved!

Years later, to this day, I have people who reach out to me after watching that talk online, letting me know they were inspired to make a change. I'm glad I didn't allow fear and doubt to keep me from giving that talk. I grew from the experience, and my mother's advice was what I leaned on when it came to future talks. Share what you know, what you've lived—no need to over-prepare—it's your story, your lived experiences. Worrying how it's received is out of my control.

I advocate that men share their health and prostate cancer experiences—including their mental health challenges and the shame that men experience. The more we share, the more we chip away and end the stigma that holds us back from being open and sharing our health issues and overcoming those challenges.

College Guys

Back in 2010, I was sitting across from Dr. Katz in his Manhattan office as he told me that decades of poor lifestyle habits were perhaps the biggest contributor to me having early-stage prostate cancer.

A little over a year later, I had a conversation with Dr. Cohen, asking his advice on what my response should be to younger men in their twenties, thirties, and forties who are reaching out to me asking if they should get a PSA test. They, like me, knew nothing about their prostates or screening for prostate cancer. I had become very aware of the controversy surrounding the PSA test and the PSA screening recommendations, which were for much older men.

Days before a man gets a PSA test, riding a bike, lifting weights, and having sex can all affect the PSA number, and that carries huge consequences. I wasn't told to abstain from those activities before my PSA. The first time I got results for a PSA, I was at the urologist getting my testosterone levels checked. That was the reason I was there. The lab had also tested PSA. Getting my PSA tested was not the reason I was there, so I wasn't told to abstain from any activities. The second PSA test I had to make sure the first one wasn't a fluke also showed a concerning high amount of PSA.

But neither time was I told to abstain from activities that could affect the number.

I've spoken with many men who also weren't told to abstain from strenuous activity before getting their PSA checked. Elevated PSA tests lead to biopsies to rule out cancer. Around 75 percent of men with an elevated PSA who get a biopsy don't have prostate cancer, which is good.[42] But unfortunately, hundreds of thousands of men had to go through an invasive, sometimes very painful procedure that, for some, can have long-term side effects. Also, there were a lot of overtreatments at the time of my diagnosis: many men diagnosed with localized slow-growing early-stage prostate cancer (a majority) were getting their prostates removed when they didn't have to, leading to many experiencing erectile dysfunction for some period, some permanently, followed by depression.

What should I tell younger men? I was grateful I caught mine when I did. And had I gone with the first doctor's recommendation, I wouldn't have a prostate. Nor would I have learned about lifestyle and be on this journey.

Dr. Cohen said the most powerful message I could share with younger men is for them to adopt healthy lifestyle habits now and understand the enormous benefits to short and long-term health. It was an empowering message that made sense to tell young men: "Here's what you can do now to reduce your risk and possibly prevent prostate cancer, along with heart disease, stroke, and diabetes."

I was having conversations every day with men of all ages about their health and their overall views on men's health issues. I was interested in learning what moved them to act, what influenced them. And I asked what they were doing to be proactive when it came to their physical and mental health needs.

When I spoke with college-aged men, I repeatedly got feedback that they didn't consider their health at all, just like me in college. A few said they were addressing men's health because they raised funds during No Shave November and Movember.

"So, you've raised funds, but what have you done for your health?" I would ask, followed by blank stares.

Many of the college-aged guys I was speaking with were overweight, some obese. More than I remember when I was in college in the '90s. What was happening? "Dad bods" were now college bods.

Young men needed to become educated on lifestyle, not become fundraisers and believe that was addressing their health, "men's health."

I asked many guys about lifestyle and cancer, and they weren't aware of a connection. Of course, they weren't. Why would I expect college guys to know that when I didn't know that at age thirty-five? They were "aware" of the words "prostate cancer" but didn't know much about it. College-aged men weren't getting PSA tests or digital rectal exams, so they had to become educated on what they could do now to prevent cancer and chronic disease. They needed to understand the consequences of poor lifestyle habits.

By sharing my story, I wanted to help men connect the dots between lifestyle habits and the risk of developing health conditions like early-stage prostate cancer, heart disease, and more. I spoke on college campuses, and afterward, when I spoke with young guys one-on-one and in small groups, they would speak with an air of invincibility, like me when I was their age. Their responses would take me back to those years of all-nighters, binge drinking, and fast food.

Not surprisingly, many would tell me they didn't know diet and lifestyle affected the risk of cancer and chronic disease. Some would share they had a father, grandfather, or uncle with prostate cancer, but more would share they had dads, uncles, and grandpas who had had a heart attack, diabetes, stroke, or other forms of cancer.

"If I had known in college what I know now," is what I thought when I heard them talk, and that's what I was trying to get these young men to understand. Now matters. Think of your family members with chronic disease and how they got there. I can draw a straight arrow to all the men in my family with poor health and their decades of unhealthy lifestyle habits.

After speaking to a large group of men at Texas A&M University (the fittest group I had spoken to), I wrote "Talking to College Guys About Cancer Prevention and Men's Health Issues" (which was published in *The Huffington Post* on 04/22/2014). Here's an excerpt of my thoughts shortly after I spoke with them.

We must do more to reach a younger generation — to educate and empower by planting seeds early in life on prevention, risk reduction and modifying unhealthy behavioral habits. We must remove the stigma and embarrassment for men to discuss their health issues and help them to become more proactive.

When I was in college I did what most college students do. I drank, partied, ate cheap fast food, and lived my college years with little regard for my future health. Planting seeds of knowledge with college students (and younger) is essential in our ongoing War on Cancer.

We shouldn't ask young men and women to serve solely as fundraisers without educating them on what they can do to reduce cancer risk, and encouraging them to learn about cancer-causing chemical exposure in the air they breathe, food they eat and personal care products they use.

After speaking to young men and women while running a cancer nonprofit, it's become clear, that if more knew they could fight cancer, before it strikes, they would do it.

Let's educate and empower our leaders of tomorrow by placing a greater focus on the causes of cancer and risk reduction — now — and not wait for what is certainly not just an old person's disease.[43]

Light It Blue / White House Blue

In August 2011, I sent out a press release with a video on how to "Go Blue" in support of September's National Prostate Cancer Awareness Month. The video started with a female voice-over sharing prostate cancer statistics that mirrored the graphics on screen, and she stated that prostate cancer "has low awareness, is underreported, underfunded, and demands more attention." I appeared in the video and let viewers know I was diagnosed with prostate cancer at age thirty-five. I then encouraged the viewer to "go blue" this September: wear a blue ribbon or a blue necktie, network blue by changing your Facebook and Twitter profile photos to a blue square, speak blue and get people talking by sharing information about prostate cancer, ask your local sports teams to wear blue bands, ask your local newspaper to write about prostate cancer in blue ink, and ask your elected officials to encourage citizens to get screenings. It continued, "Ask your mayor to light up City Hall blue, ask the White House to light it blue one night in September." I end the video by speaking into the camera and saying, "Awareness will lead to action, and action will save lives." Soon after I released the video, Houston Mayor Annise Parker lit City Hall blue for a week, and Blue Cure received a mayoral proclamation.

I was trying. I simply felt prostate cancer and men's health issues weren't getting anywhere near the attention women's health issues received.

Years before, I saw news coverage of President George W. Bush lighting the White House pink, and across Houston, buildings lit pink in observance of breast cancer awareness in October. But no blue White House.

I wanted to see buildings across America lit blue. I wanted blue to stand for more than the words "prostate cancer." I wanted "action" to be associated with prostate cancer, and that meant scheduling a checkup and a prostate cancer screening and adopting healthy lifestyle habits. I didn't understand why buildings across America and the world were not lit blue in September but lit pink every October for Breast Cancer Awareness Month. I was asked this question repeatedly by wives, daughters, and sisters, "Why so much pink but no blue for our men?"

Every year after 2011, I emailed, posted, tweeted, and called on elected officials and business leaders to light their buildings and landmarks blue for one evening during September's National Prostate Cancer Awareness Month. Every year, I saw more buildings lit blue.

In 2014, six years after President George W. Bush started the annual tradition of lighting the White House pink during October's Breast Cancer Awareness Month, I continued to ask why the White House wasn't being lit blue in observance of prostate cancer awareness or men's health? I felt it was overdue for the "People's House" to be lit blue in recognition of the most commonly diagnosed men's cancer in America.

During the Obama administration, We the People was an online platform that allowed Americans to create a petition that would receive an official response from the administration if the petition received 100,000 online signatures. I saw the We the People petition as an opportunity to light the White House blue, and that would get our lifestyle message out there. Reaching that 100,000-signature benchmark became my goal. In June 2014, during Men's Health Month, I started a campaign in support of the petition. I produced a video of a young mother speaking into the camera, calling for the White House to be lit blue for her son, her husband, and the men in her life. I was interviewed about the campaign and the petition on various television networks and in print and online media. I wrote about why I was launching this campaign and its importance, and I heavily pushed it on social media. Influencers got behind the campaign: many of the NFL Houston Texans, some elected congress people and mayors and celebrities like Kelly Clarkson, Sophia Bush, Bun B, the Backstreet Boys, Seth Rogen, Drew Rosenhaus, Matt Leinart, Duane Brown, Chris Myers, Connor Barwin, Jenny Johnson, Sheila Jackson Lee, Pete Olson, Fran Drescher, Hall of Fame Quarterback Warren Moon, Owen Daniels, Weird Al Yankovic, the NFL Players Association, urologists, health-care professionals, and prostate cancer survivors and supporters signed the petition and publicly shared on social media with the hashtags #WhiteHouseBlue and #SignforDad. Most of the celebrities who took to Twitter to encourage their supporters to sign the petition were friends of Jenny Johnson, a comedian and writer who lost her father to prostate cancer and had joined Blue Cure's board of directors.

The petition received millions of media and social media impressions, but disappointingly, those impressions and eyeballs didn't translate to online signatures. The petition only received a few thousand signatures. It stung. Did people not care? I was at a loss.

After a week of reflection, I looked at the positive. I considered the millions of media impressions that resulted and believed there was a ripple effect that would result in men, some fathers and grandfathers, scheduling an annual checkup or a prostate cancer screening, and some would adopt healthier lifestyle habits. I looked at the entire experience as a learning experience to build on.

The next year, the Light it Blue—#LightitBlue—campaign would try a different strategy, more grassroots, developing graphics and scripts for supporters to post on social media and share with friends. A college intern helped build and compile databases of the top one hundred city halls and fifty state capitols, major hospitals and cancer centers, arenas and stadiums, landmarks and monuments. We sent hundreds of emails and followed up with hundreds of calls, leaving messages. We were persistent. It was ground-level grassroots.

I again wrote about the reasons for the campaign and published pieces in *The Huffington Post* and the *Houston Chronicle,* and I did broadcast television interviews. Major cancer centers such as Dana-Farber in Boston, the Seattle Cancer Care Alliance/Fred Hutch in Seattle, Baylor College of Medicine in Houston lit blue, and others soon followed. We began to see landmarks, hospitals, more city halls illuminated and acknowledge lighting blue for prostate cancer, prevention, and men's health.

After years of grassroots campaigning, emails, phone calls, social media, enlisting celebrities, writing byline articles and media interviews, a very large research-focused prostate cancer nonprofit with deep pockets adopted the #LightitBlue hashtag, proclaimed they were lighting buildings across America blue, and began fundraising off the Light it Blue campaign. I had people reach out to me asking if we had partnered. No, I would have, but they didn't reach out to me. They didn't acknowledge our hard work and impact, nor was lifestyle part of their campaign. Their big budget got behind the campaign, claimed it as their own, and raised money. It is what it is...(sigh) nonprofits. At the end of the day, I hope they raised more money for research that, hopefully, one day, gets us closer to a medical cure.

CHAPTER FOURTEEN

LECTURE SERIES

The holistic, whole-body approach I adopted in managing my early-stage prostate cancer had the benefits of preventing, reducing the risk, and reversing various chronic diseases that are leading killers of men. This was *the* vital message for Blue Cure to advocate and share, which is why when I developed the Blue Cure Lecture Series, I envisioned speakers that would deliver that message. Carolyn Farb would turn that vision into reality. She first approached Board Member Jim McClellan to be the major underwriter to get the Lecture Series off the ground. He saw its importance and agreed, and without his generous support, the Lecture Series wouldn't have happened.

Carolyn wasn't afraid to ask, and she repeatedly told me when you believe, you can bring needed change by asking for the resources to make it happen. Don't be afraid to ask. Just ask.

Margaret Cuomo

After my prostate cancer diagnosis, I developed a growing curiosity about the effects of chemicals in our environment, and the products we use on our body, in our homes, and on our lawn.

During my research, I read the President's Cancer Panel, 2008–2009 Annual Report, excerpts in the following letter to President Barack Obama:

"The panel urges you most strongly to use the power of your office to remove the carcinogens and other toxins from our food, water, and air that needlessly increase healthcare costs, cripple our nation's productivity, and devastate American lives.'

'...the true burden of environmentally induced cancer has been grossly underestimated. With nearly 80,000 chemicals on the market in the United States, many of which are used by millions of Americans in their daily lives and are un- or understudied and largely unregulated, exposure to potential environmental carcinogens is widespread.

"With the growing body of evidence linking environmental exposures to cancer, the public is becoming increasingly aware of the unacceptable burden of cancer resulting from environmental and occupational exposures that could have been prevented through appropriate national action"[44]

I read about American veterans who fought in Vietnam who were exposed to Agent Orange and, decades later, developed prostate cancer. I questioned how that could happen and learned that a carcinogen is any substance or agent that causes cancer, and this can happen by inhalation, absorption on skin, and digestion. That intrigued me. Was the link between Agent Orange and prostate cancer a result of inhalation—the air they were breathing while in Vietnam—absorption of the chemical on their skin, or digestion from the chemical being sprayed on food troops consumed? Or all the above? Learning about Agent Orange and environmental exposure and cancer being underestimated, it had me ponder the effects of decades of cumulative exposures from other chemicals in the air I breathe (Houston, Texas, has some of the worst air quality), the chemicals in and on the food I eat, the chemicals in household cleaning products, lawn-care products, and products I use on my body.

I thought of the testosterone gel I rubbed on my shoulder before my diagnosis and how quickly my testosterone levels increased, my energy and muscle mass increased, and my body fat decreased. My skin absorbing the little bit of gel I rubbed on my shoulder had a drastic effect on my body.

I believe that there were ingredients in the gel that allowed for the testosterone supplement to work the way it did. And not being a chemist or scientist, I didn't know how it worked, but the testosterone gel was my frame of reference. As was the medication I applied on my face and scalp for decades that helped the symptoms of my seborrheic dermatitis, which caused itchiness, flakiness, and redness on my scalp, hairline, and around my nostrils.

My dermatologists were never able to answer me when I asked what the causes of my seborrheic dermatitis were. But over the years, I took many prescription medications with different active ingredients to manage the symptoms. So, the intended effect of what I was applying on my face and scalp was to help in a positive way, but I wondered what ingredients my skin was absorbing that could have long-term harmful effects.

The testosterone gel and medications I used on my face and scalp are examples that were my frame of reference that what I applied on my skin influenced my body, from my hormones to reducing inflammation and improving my appearance.

What about my decades of use of sunscreens, antiperspirants, deodorants, moisturizers, and toothpaste? Every day I used those products, and not once did I read their ingredients. Were they all healthy? We all assume if it's on a grocery or pharmacy shelf, it's been tested and is safe. Right? Were there long-term effects? I wasn't trying to be a hypochondriac. I was searching high and low for answers for my prostate cancer diagnosis.

The seed was planted when I learned about Agent Orange and prostate cancer. I continued to seek information, and my interest grew when I read Dr. David Servan-Schreiber's book *Anticancer* and watched some of his interviews about avoiding toxins in household cleaners and body care products.

I tried to share a lot of what I was learning on social media. I received messages of interest, with many letting me know they had never thought of possible cancer-causing effects from the chemicals in our air, water, food, household, and body care products.

I read a story in *The Daily Beast* called "Are We Wasting Billions Seeking a Cure for Cancer?" The provocative headline caught my attention. It was an article adapted from Margaret I. Cuomo's book, *A World Without Cancer*.

The article argued for more funding and resources for cancer prevention research and initiatives to make an immediate impact.

> "...we have not adequately channeled our scientific know-how, funding, and energy into a full exploration of the one path certain to save lives: prevention. That it should become the ultimate goal of cancer research has been recognized since the war on cancer began.
>
> It is time to commit our resources to more aggressively studying the ways in which diet, exercise, supplements, environmental exposure, and other factors can influence the development of cancer."[45]

So many points about this excerpt struck a chord with me and what I was learning. She was addressing "cancer prevention," which so many were telling me wasn't possible. I immediately ordered *A World Without Cancer*, read it a few times, and focused more on why government agencies, non-profits, and health-care entities weren't placing a greater focus and funding on cancer prevention strategies.

Margaret's MD credential carried weight, which is why I posted about *A World Without Cancer* on social media. I wanted the doubters, including an MD who told me cancer could not be prevented, to know about Margaret's book. It was important to draw attention to the topic of lifestyle and cancer prevention and get answers, and for the public to gain knowledge to reduce our cancer risk and cancer burden. Many cancer survivors I spoke with told me, "My doctor never told me about diet or environmental exposures, so I don't believe it." This is what I mostly heard as I met men going through prostate cancer treatment. I shared how I had changed my dietary and lifestyle habits. Oftentimes, because their doctors never discussed diet and lifestyle, they dismissed Blue Cure and what it was advocating.

I wanted Blue Cure to align with experts like Margaret. I wanted to meet her, let her know my story, Blue Cure's mission, how I was using it to change the way men look at prostate cancer and their health, and discuss ways we could partner. I wanted to introduce her message to the prostate cancer and men's health community I was fostering. I wanted men to be proactive and become educated on the root causes of cancer: diet, lifestyle, pollutants, harmful and questionable chemicals in household, personal hygiene, and lawn care products.

I finally met with Carolyn Farb over lunch and shared what I had learned from *A World Without Cancer*. I asked for suggestions on ways Blue Cure could partner with Dr. Cuomo to share and amplify her message. I wanted some out-of-the-box ideas before I contacted Dr. Cuomo, which is what I planned. Carolyn's eyebrow raised, "Invite Margaret to be a keynote speaker at the inaugural Blue Cure Lecture Series."

Lecture series? I stared at her, digesting what she just said. She continued, "Blue Cure needs to have a speakers series with keynote addresses from these experts you speak of that research lifestyle, environment, diet, and effects on our health and cancer."

I nodded in agreement and smiled, "Absolutely, Carolyn. I'll reach out to Margaret and see how we can get her to Houston to speak at our event."

"It will happen." Carolyn said as we continued the conversation walking to her home office. Carolyn handed me a stack of invitations and programs from previous events she had supported and chaired. She told me to peruse them later and become familiar with the benefactors. We began brainstorming ideas and writing a to-do list. Carolyn would put her full support behind this event to add credibility to our organization and mission. She believed in the message.

The next day, I contacted Dr. Cuomo. I shared my story, my admiration of her work, and my strong interest in having her speak in Houston at the Blue Cure Lecture Series. I asked if we could meet in person in the next few months, and Dr. Cuomo agreed.

On January 15, 2013, at Dr. Cuomo's suggestion, we met at Rouge Tomate in Chelsea, Manhattan, a plant-centered restaurant with a variety of healthy options.

Dr. Cuomo ate a plant-based lunch and expounded on her views from *A World Without Cancer*. She answered all my questions, asked about my life, my experiences meeting with the various doctors, how I handled varying medical opinions, my mental health, and the emotional ups and downs. Every question she asked got me to open up and share. She listened and appeared genuinely interested.

She praised the mission of Blue Cure and how I was sharing my story to raise awareness about lifestyle and prostate cancer and how I was using social media to connect. Dr. Cuomo recognized the stigma men have in confronting health-care needs and was encouraging upon hearing that Blue Cure was enlisting professional athletes to help spread the message of prevention and healthy lifestyles.

I told her why I wanted her to be our inaugural speaker. Her message would be illuminating to people in that ballroom: Houston's business leaders, influencers, doctors, supporters, and members of media. They needed to hear it. I didn't care if what she said could make them uncomfortable. Margaret speaking at our event would help define to others what Blue Cure was about.

Her parting words were to "fight the good fight and stay the course… men, younger men, need to hear this message."

I wrote about our two-hour lunch in the *Houston Chronicle* (Jan 16, 2013):

> Dr. Cuomo has a deeply instilled commitment and service to others, which was immediately evident during our lunch. She repeatedly expressed a need to change the status quo so we can prevent cancer and save lives. After more than 40 years and $90 billion-plus dollars spent on the "War on Cancer," cancer still kills over 1,500 Americans daily and there's still no cure. This deeply troubles Dr. Cuomo, who says we cannot accept this as our new normal.

Over the next few hours, we discussed some of the startling facts presented in *A World Without Cancer*, such as:[46]

- Cancer is responsible for one in four deaths in America.
- Research shows that we can prevent half of all cancer with what we know now.
- The National Cancer Institute spends $3.3 billion on research for cancer treatment vs. only $232 million for prevention.
- Tobacco companies spend $10 billion a year to market cancer-causing cigarettes in the U.S.
- Obesity, poor diet, and lack of exercise account for 30 percent of all cancers.
- Many simple steps, such as eating cooked red tomatoes and adding the spice turmeric to food, can cut the risk of cancer.
- Despite the fact that heavy people are more than 50 percent more likely to die from cancer than normal-weight people, the government still grants more federal subsidies for corn-based additives such as high fructose corn syrup and cornstarch than it does for healthier fruits and green vegetables.
- The proper amount of Vitamin D can reduce the risk of many cancers, including colon, breast, ovarian and prostate cancers, but the federal government and public health officials are not doing enough to promote its benefits.
- More than 400 chemicals that are suspected or proven carcinogens (any substance causing cancer) are commonly found in our food, water, and air.
- Bisphenol A (BPA), a chemical commonly found in many plastics, canned food and other items, has been linked to breast cancer, prostate cancer, diabetes and hyperactivity and aggression in children. Studies show that parabens may stimulate the growth of hormone related cancers, and traces of the preservative have been found in breast tumors. Yet parabens are widely found in popular cosmetics, moisturizers, and

hair products. The FDA should ban the use of these harmful chemicals in consumer products.

Later that year, on September 27, 2013, Margaret came down to Houston as the speaker at the inaugural Blue Cure Lecture Series Luncheon. We also honored former Houston superintendent and our seventh United States secretary of education, prostate cancer survivor, Dr. Rod Paige for his service to our country and his prostate cancer patient advocacy. Former US President George W. Bush sent a letter that was read aloud by Carolyn Farb in tribute to Dr. Paige. In his message, President Bush also thanked everyone for their efforts to increase prostate cancer awareness and prevention and promote healthy living.

Dr. Cuomo presented the data and key points from her book and ways we each can live healthier and happier lives by taking simple actions each day that can lower our risk for cancer. These include choosing healthy foods, keeping physically and mentally active, avoiding harmful chemicals in household and personal care products, ending smoking, and managing stress.

Dr. Cuomo received a long-standing ovation when she concluded her talk. Her presentation had eye-opening data that didn't mask the current reality of America's health-care dilemma. But Dr. Cuomo's message was hopeful, urging every attendee that we have a lot of opportunity and power with our choices, to prevent and reduce our cancer risk.

The event was on the local evening NBC news, in the local papers, and received some national media. I co-chaired the event with Carolyn, but 99.9 percent of it was all her. She made it all happen, and I learned by watching her. Carolyn spent literally hundreds of hours writing hundreds of personalized emails, cultivating prospective benefactors, setting up the silent and live auctions, creating the event program, the menu, Dr. Cuomo's accommodations. … Carolyn pretty much did everything. Again, Carolyn's "magic" was the behind-the-scenes work most don't see, and her volunteerism continued to show me how much she believed in Blue Cure.

The feedback from attendees was positive—much of it letting me know the luncheon and Margaret's speech gave them a lot to think about. It's something when you hear that from urologists.

John Mackey – November 6, 2014

I watched an interview with Whole Foods Market founder and CEO John Mackey and learned that he believed a whole-foods plant-based diet could prevent many chronic diseases and cancers killing Americans. After watching that interview, I wanted to meet him. I asked my board members if anyone knew John Mackey or an executive at Whole Foods Market, because John should know about Blue Cure and help us spread our message. Perhaps Whole Foods Market could sponsor one of our lifestyle education programs. Despite each of my board members being seemingly connected to everyone, from Hollywood celebrities and professional athletes to elected leaders and former US presidents, no one knew John Mackey or anyone who was acquainted with him.

Literally the following week, on November 6, 2014, I was picking up a suit being altered, but when I got to the store, it wasn't ready. So I decided to go next door and grab a bite at a new Whole Foods Market celebrating its grand opening. It was packed. Luckily, I found a seat in the crowded dining area. My eyes locked on a recognizable face seated maybe twenty feet away, but I couldn't place a name with the face. I worked on my salad a little more and looked up again, and that's when it hit me. Seated across from me was John Mackey. He was engaged in a conversation with someone. Could have been an executive, a buyer, a vendor, a friend. I had to interrupt, but how without appearing rude? A few minutes later, John got up to take a call on his mobile, and I approached the person he was speaking with and asked if she would mind if I said hello to John. She grudgingly nodded okay and told me to make it quick.

As John got off his call, I went up to him, my arm extended for a handshake, introduced myself, and told him I was a fan of what he had built and the values Whole Foods Market represented. He stared at me and looked over at the lady waiting on him. He shook my hand, thanked me, and began to walk back towards the person waiting on him. I mentioned I had prostate cancer and asked him about speaking at a Blue Cure event, and he interrupted me and said he had a speaking fee, it goes to charity, and I would need to contact his representatives and discuss. As if I didn't hear what he just told me, I proceeded to give a shortened version of my TED Talk, "Changing the Way We Fight Cancer," and he actually stood there listening until I finished. I strongly made my point that men in America were dying prematurely and needed to hear a message of lifestyle and prevention.

John had a smirk, "You're very passionate. I agree with what you said. I'm going to give you the email to my assistant. We will do something." I tried to play it cool, but my facial expressions probably betrayed me with a big goofy grin. Just a week earlier, I had been asking my board members if they knew John or someone who did, and there we were shaking hands, with him telling me, "We will do something."

Where would it lead?

That evening, I emailed his assistant. We spoke by phone a few days later, and I told her I was inquiring about John speaking at the Blue Cure Lecture Series. Is that something I would need to speak with his agent about? Since we are a nonprofit, would they be able to offer us a reduced fee? A week went by, then two weeks. Was he not interested? By this point, I had told Carolyn and my board about the meeting with John and was waiting on a response. My hope was John would offer us a reduced speaking fee, but Carolyn had already begun to reach out to benefactors to secure an underwriter. With Carolyn by my side and in my corner, she would make it happen. I wanted to have John speak. A successful businessman who believed in a message I was advocating, sharing how lifestyle helped him be a leader and could help solve America's broken health-care system. It was important for men to hear this and for Blue Cure to continue to be positioned as an organization focusing on men's health and root causes and prevention. I know not all cancer cases can be prevented, but most can, as can many chronic diseases. And that's a message that most men aren't aware of. I was working to change that.

I heard back from John's assistant that he would speak at the Blue Cure Lecture Series, and to my great surprise, John would waive his speaking fee. I didn't expect that. I didn't know if John saw the link of TV interviews I sent his assistant or my TED Talk, but his accepting my invitation to speak and waiving his speaking fee was a big boost of confidence and validation.

Since John would be coming from Austin to Houston, I told his assistant we would take care of his travel and hotel. She told me not to worry about it. John would take care of his accommodations. He was happy to come speak and support Blue Cure.

On March 26, 2015, John delivered his highly anticipated talk to a packed ballroom of 450 attendees: business and community leaders, philanthropists, professional athletes, doctors, and members of the media. Most were friends of Carolyn Farb's who purchased seats and tables to support a cause she believed in, and many were there believing they would hear an American business success story. From the reactions, I don't think that many expected to hear the kind of hard-hitting speech on lifestyle they got.

Leading up to John's speech, I had watched every interview of him discussing the role of diet and disease. John didn't mince words. He presented data and his views, and his delivery wasn't soft. I kind of knew what to expect but wasn't sure how the audience of meat-eating oil executives and Houston's philanthropy set would take it. It is Houston, Texas, a foodie capital, where Mexican and steak restaurants reign supreme—and so does obesity.

John presented a lot of data that showed how, over the decades, America's dietary habits increased to more processed foods and high-fat animal foods. Our waistlines went up, and so did preventable chronic health conditions and cancer rates. John's talk was a hard-hitting presentation, and it was met with loud groans. I looked around, and many were shaking their head in disapproval. Some were booing, and others had completely tuned out and were talking to others at their table. John heard the grumbling and said, "I think I've lost a lot of you." He did. It's not what they had expected, and they didn't want to hear it. For a second, I felt bad for John and what it meant for Blue Cure, but I believed in everything he was saying. I realized it had to happen. People had to hear the uncomfortable truth. We could have offered attendees a high-fat, high sugar menu and provided some sort of entertainment to raise funds in support of research. We could have avoided mentioning the root causes and prevention and telling attendees that they needed to accept a level of responsibility, take account of their lifestyle habits, and make changes. But that was not the message John gave, and that's not why I started Blue Cure.

I was asked afterward if I regretted inviting John. "Not at all. Sometimes the truth hurts."

Dean Ornish, MD – April 12, 2016

In between visiting various urologists, I read about Dr. Dean Ornish's research on heart disease and prostate cancer. It took that first year of my journey—visiting Dr. Katz and going on active holistic surveillance, meeting the then-president of MD Anderson Cancer Center, Dr. Mendelsohn, reading *Anticancer* by David Servan-Schreiber, corresponding with Dr. Lorenzo Cohen, and, finally, Dr. Cohen's encouragement to read Dean Ornish's research on prostate cancer—for me to truly understand the significance of Dr. Ornish's research on lifestyle changes and a low-fat vegan diet for heart disease prevention and reversal and for slowing the progression of early-stage prostate cancer.

The more I read about Dr. Ornish's work and the more interviews of him I watched, the more I asked why more urologists weren't sharing the findings of his research, urging their patients to change their lifestyle habits. Why was it that 100 percent of the men with prostate cancer I had met had not been counseled on diet and lifestyle?

Dr. Ornish's research on early-stage prostate cancer was published in 2005, five years before my diagnosis. Yet years after my diagnosis, I continued to meet men with prostate cancer who said they received no counsel on lifestyle and dietary changes. It blew me away.

I wanted to call attention to Dr. Ornish's research and invite him to speak at the Blue Cure Lecture Series. Our Facebook following was approaching 200,000, and promoting the event would include lots of education to our community on social media, writing byline articles, and pitching pre- and post-event coverage to various media outlets. I also knew urologists would be aware of what Blue Cure was promoting, and I wanted them to investigate Dr. Ornish's research findings and counsel their patients or refer their patients to a dietitian.

I had dinner with Carolyn Farb, telling her I wanted us to get Dr. Ornish as our next speaker for the Blue Cure Lecture Series. He's the "father of lifestyle medicine," and I wanted everyone Blue Cure touched to know that I still lived with early-stage prostate cancer and that Dr. Ornish's research gave me hope; that it's the reason I believe in the power of lifestyle changes.

She was very supportive and told me her good friends Barbara and Gerald Hines were personal friends and supporters of Dr. Ornish. Decades earlier, Gerald Hines, the world-renowned famed real estate developer, helped fund some of Dr. Ornish's lifestyle medicine research.

After Carolyn spoke with Barbara and Gerald Hines about Dr. Ornish, they personally reached out and asked him if he would speak at the Blue Cure Lecture Series. He accepted.

The event was chaired by former NFL players Chris Myers and Ryan Pontbriand, who were on Blue Cure's board of directors. Their involvement brought to our event a few handfuls of NFL players and professional athletes. I loved that Blue Cure had a growing association with professional athletes. Most perceive professional athletes as hyper-masculine dudes who are big carnivores. Blue Cure didn't shy away from promoting whole-foods plant-based nutrition. We always have, and that's not the association expected with big, burly jocks. These athletes weren't vegan, but they agreed men need to eat more plants!

Also in attendance from Los Angeles was comedian and Blue Cure Board Member Jenny Johnson, who had been responsible for getting a large group of celebrities to support the effort to light The White House blue. She brought along her friends rapper Bun-B, country music artist Rich O' Toole, and some others. It was an eclectic crowd. I was pumped to have attracted such a diverse audience of influencers who would take to social media. I knew their presence would help us garner additional media coverage about our event and Dr. Ornish's research on lifestyle interventions for heart disease and prostate cancer. Dr. Ornish was scheduled for twenty-five minutes, but he spoke for close to an hour. I had seen so many of his speeches on YouTube that I knew what he would say and how he would say it. But I was still riveted. I looked around the ballroom and saw everyone giving him their full attention. He boiled down his research findings to say it's all about lifestyle: eat more plants, move more, stress less, and love more.

Erin Brockovich

In 2000, I watched *Erin Brockovich*, the movie starring Julia Roberts (who won an Academy Award for her role) that was based on the true story of a scrappy unemployed single mother of three who discovers a cover-up involving a cancer-causing chemical in the water supply sickening the residents of Hinkley, California. Erin is a no-bullshit crusader whose persistence in uncovering the truth helped the "powerless and voiceless" take on a powerful corporation and win. It was David vs. Goliath. Erin's hard work and determination were instrumental in winning the largest settlement ever awarded at the time for a direct-action lawsuit against Pacific Gas & Electric. One takeaway from her story that made an impression on me is there are companies and executives that will lie at the expense of consumer health and safety to protect their bottom line.

My prostate cancer led to my growing curiosity about chemical exposures and cancer. Before my diagnosis, I couldn't care less. I wasn't concerned about pollutants in the air I breathed or the chemicals in the products I used. I didn't read labels. But everything came into question after my diagnosis when I read that only 5 to 10 percent of prostate cancers were due to inherited genetic mutations. Ninety to ninety-five percent weren't, and I was learning diet, lifestyle, and environmental exposures were big factors.

Most eye-opening and troubling was reading the 2008–2009 Annual Report from the President's Cancer Panel titled *Reducing Environmental Cancer Risk: What We Can Do Now*. This led to more questions and a need for answers. I read this report shortly after my diagnosis.

> (Excerpt) "With the growing body of evidence linking environmental exposures to cancer, the public is becoming increasingly aware of the unacceptable burden of cancer resulting from environmental and occupational exposures that could have been prevented through appropriate national action.

Research on environmental causes of cancer has been limited by low priority and inadequate funding…

The Panel was particularly concerned to find that the true burden of environmentally induced cancer has been grossly underestimated. With nearly 80,000 chemicals on the market in the United States, many of which are used by millions of Americans in their daily lives and are un- or understudied and largely unregulated, exposure to potential environmental carcinogens is widespread. One such ubiquitous chemical, bisphenol A (BPA), is still found in many consumer products and remains unregulated in the United States, despite the growing link between BPA and several diseases, including various cancers."[47]

I wondered why more wasn't known. Why was there "inadequate funding" on environmental causes and cancer? Did the special interest money that funds the campaigns of elected leaders come at the expense of our health and safety by influencing them to not impose regulation that protects Americans? We needed more focus on environmental causes and cancer. We needed answers and solutions.

I've been asking these questions and raising these issues about the link between our environment and cancer since I started the Journey with Prostate Cancer Facebook page in 2010. I've had numerous conversations with men, and not surprisingly, they have little to no knowledge about environmental exposures and cancer. Most don't know about endocrine-disrupting chemicals, how ubiquitous they are, and the potential harms they pose. Most men I've talked to tell me they don't read labels on food products, deodorant, sunscreen, and weed killer. Many honestly believe these products wouldn't be on the market if they were harmful.

I wanted to inspire curiosity in men to have a greater interest in the chemicals that inundate us every day and the cumulative effect they have on our health. By becoming educated, men can make choices that are healthier and safer. The more men gain knowledge, the need for answers grows, and the call for change becomes louder and within reach. That's my hope. But, simply, men don't know.

Blue Cure had focused a lot on diet and lifestyle, but I wanted to give greater attention to our environment and cancer, and that's why I asked Erin Brockovich to speak at our Lecture Series. Erin's presence would remind our community about her story and call attention to the ubiquity of harmful and questionable chemicals all around us by starting with the one thing we all use and need for survival: water.

Eighteen years after watching *Erin Brockovich*, I flew out to Los Angeles to meet Erin for lunch at a hotel in Beverly Hills, California. I wanted to get to know her and write about our conversation for a series of articles and social media posts to generate interest in her upcoming talk at the Blue Cure Lecture Series. We needed all the promotion and publicity we could get to sell tickets since we had to reschedule Erin's first appearance due to Hurricane Harvey, which devastated Houston, and us.

I waited in the dining area overlooking the garden courtyard at the Montage Hotel. I wasn't sure if Erin would be coming with a publicist or an assistant. I didn't know what to expect, but I had an hour of her time and was interested in getting to know her and finding out if her personality was as big as Julia Roberts' Oscar-winning performance.

She didn't disappoint. I heard her before I saw her. Erin shouted, "Hey!" when she entered the dining area. I looked up and saw her with her distressed jeans tucked into her knee-high fitted black boots, black top, big black sunglasses, and her long blonde hair pulled back. She looked like a celebrity. I don't know why I had this image of her coming in business meeting attire. As I stood to greet her, she vented about the "shitty" traffic she was stuck in and apologized for being a few minutes late. I hadn't noticed. She sat down, and we began talking like we knew each other. She seemed comfortable and spoke with no filter, colorfully making her points with expletives—a "fuck" here, a "fuck" there. She gave me a mini-education on municipal water systems, how no two bodies of water are identical—like fingerprints—how different water is from one municipality to the next, how water is cleaned and treated, how there are unsafe levels of contaminants linked to cancer and other health issues in water, what can be done, and the need for action. I knew a lot of what she was sharing from my research, but listening to her share stories and express her thoughts allowed me to feel her passion and see up close her determination and grit. Our scheduled one-hour meeting went over two hours, and there was never a lull. I was moved and inspired when we finished our meeting. I called Carolyn when the meeting was over and said, "There's a reason there was a movie made about her. I've never met anyone like her."

I couldn't wait to have her speak in Houston.

On May 11, 2018, Erin spoke at the Blue Cure Lecture Series and captivated a packed ballroom. She was personal, sharing revealing stories about her life experiences, which led to her passion to help people and her life's work in consumer advocacy and environmental activism. Her vulnerability wasn't something we had seen before from any of our previous speakers. She connected with the audience and drew them in, and when Erin got to the meat of her talk about chemicals in our water, everyone was 100 percent locked in. I looked around: no one was disengaged or checking their phone. They were focused on Erin. She presented accompanying slides with data, charts, and graphs, and she encouraged action to all in attendance. But her authenticity and masterful storytelling had me and the audience hanging on her every word. It's why when she finished, she was met with thunderous applause and the longest standing ovation of any of our speakers.

I told our audience the inspiration and motivation from Erin's talk had to move us to act. Let's not let the chemicals in our water be the endpoint of our consumer advocacy and environmental activism. Let it be the starting point that moves us to question the chemicals in our environment and in the products that we use every day in our lives—because our health depends on it.

Erin had to get to the airport to make a scheduled flight, but a lot of the audience stayed around, clamoring to meet her. She stayed till every person who waited to say hello got to meet her, and she took photos with every person that asked. I walked Erin to a waiting car and thanked her again. I let her know how moved I was and that we had just experienced a rock-star moment in the ballroom inside the Hilton. She thanked me for having her, turned to me, and looked me in the eyes, sharing some words of encouragement to keep fighting for truth and to continue to help others. We embraced.

Erin Brockovich's appearance at the Blue Cure Lecture Series received a tremendous amount of positive feedback and had many asking about our next guest speaker. I was happy to secure two bestselling authors and renowned physicians as speakers for the 2020 and 2021 Blue Cure Lecture Series. Unfortunately, COVID-19 happened, and we couldn't have either event. There is a silver lining. For years, I had been encouraged to host a podcast. Not knowing when we would be able to resume the Lecture Series, I decided to launch the Blue Cure Men's Health podcast. This podcast would allow me to interview leading experts on all aspects of men's physical and mental health, with lifestyle and prevention being a focus of every discussion. The response has been great, and we're able to reach more men with relevant health-promoting content each week.

The Blue Cure Lecture Series will return one day. It's an important fundraiser that supports our men's health prevention education and awareness programs. But now, the bestselling authors and physicians I would seek out for the Lecture Series are accessible and available to anyone via the Blue Cure Men's Health Podcast. It's an efficient way to learn and apply knowledge.

CHAPTER FIFTEEN
SIGNS ACROSS AMERICA

Driving for Men's Health and Leaning into Prevention

An 8,867-mile road trip around America in 2019 would be a defining chapter in my decade living with prostate cancer. It would provide clarity for the direction of my advocacy and the direction I'd take Blue Cure. In short, the experience of the trip had me recognize I must lean into prevention and do so unapologetically.

Doubting My Beliefs and Changing the Mission?

A year earlier, the Blue Cure board members and I sat through a presentation led by a group of executive MBA graduates from a prestigious university. Blue Cure had been one of the nonprofits awarded a strategic plan developed by a team of business executives. We were told the in-kind "value" of their time to develop the plan amounted to over $100,000. Seemed impressive. The board was hopeful when we began the process, believing their fresh perspective and diverse business backgrounds would provide a solution to the challenges that we experienced in identifying funding sources for prevention education programs.

Months later, we sat quietly digesting their findings and recommendations presented on a bunch of PowerPoint slides. It wasn't what any of us expected. They recommended that Blue Cure pivot from lifestyle and prevention advocacy and education to instead focus on raising funds for research for a cure to end prostate cancer. Their analysis was that the elusive big donor dollars and pharma sponsorships would come if we changed our mission to focus on research. I countered that there were already numerous cancer nonprofits and cancer centers raising money for prostate cancer research.

I was frustrated. The team interviewed me multiple times and knew exactly why I started Blue Cure. It wasn't to replicate other organizations whose main mission was to fund research for a medical cure. I would have joined the fundraising efforts of those nonprofit organizations, but that's not the need that wasn't being met. It was my story as a thirty-five-year-old diagnosed with prostate cancer and lack of knowledge on the effects of an individual's lifestyle that led me to start Blue Cure. That message wasn't out there. There were already many organizations raising hundreds of millions annually for cancer research. I reminded them that since Nixon signed the National Cancer Act in 1971, more than $100 billion had been spent on research, and billions of dollars are allocated to the NCI and other programs annually by Congress. Raising funds for research is already in place, and there are numerous groups that lobby Congress for increased funding. But what is severely lacking is attention, advocacy, and education on prevention, which is empowering and can save lives now. They acknowledged that but insisted the funding was greater if we focused on medical research. We could continue to advocate for lifestyle changes, but they recommended that not be our core focus. That's not where the funding opportunities are.

I thanked them for their months of research, but it didn't feel right. It felt like I was giving in, being told what I had created and worked hard on wasn't meaningful or relevant and wasn't making an impact. It was. But I just couldn't get the funding to do it the way I wanted to do it. I questioned whether the consultants ever really understood Blue Cure's mission— whether they understood me—and my reason for starting the organization. Through the numerous conversations I had with each team member, I knew none of them personally lived the lifestyle I advocated. How could their lifestyle habits not have influenced their approach to the project? It's the same with how doctors treat patients. The many overweight and obese urologists and primary care physicians I've spoken with about lifestyle pay it no attention.

However, because our team of consultants consisted of successful business leaders with executive MBAs, I reluctantly went along, allowing myself to believe they must know more than me. I shouldn't have. I had had my boots on the ground, talking in person and online to tens of thousands of men and family members since my diagnosis in 2010. I knew what messaging was lacking and what was missing. I believed it was why men were dying prematurely and receiving prostate cancer diagnoses at an advanced stage. I reluctantly went along with the recommendation of the consultants. But it didn't feel right, and it would be short-lived. It was a letdown.

To be clear, I support medical research and continue to hope and pray for a medical cure for metastatic prostate cancer and for new treatments that allow men to live longer and enjoy a relatively good quality of life. They can't come soon enough. The year of my diagnosis, I was told we were close to a cure. Every year since, I've read we are close. Maybe tomorrow we will have a cure, but until then, there's a need and great purpose for the empowering message I've been advocating. It's a message that could save lives now.

Over the years, I felt like I had been beaten down over and over by one "highly recommended" nonprofit fundraising consultant after another. Each time, when I shared my story and why I started Blue Cure, I was met with blank stares and "hmmm's." I received recommendations encouraging us to pivot from lifestyle and prevention to raising funds for medical research. Consultants would suggest we work with sponsors that didn't align with our message, like an alcoholic distributor or food product that wanted to plaster their signage all over one of our events. It's like these nonprofit consultants weren't listening when I shared why I started Blue Cure and how I was using it to change health messaging to men. I was talking to a wall.

There were fundraising suggestions for Blue Cure to get a percentage of sales by promoting "Cupcakes for a Cure" and similar fundraising gimmicks with pizzas, hot dogs, hamburgers, barbecue, you name it.... And every single time, I would explain again why it wasn't a fit and how it would be perceived I was promoting those foods or brands just so we could get 10 to 15 percent of net sales donated back to Blue Cure. It would always be brought to my attention that such and such cancer nonprofit or cancer center partners with those brands and food products. They were right. They did. What kind of message did that send to men and families? That those foods can't be bad, or rather, perhaps they're good for you! Almost every consultant I met with had one thing in common: each was overweight or obese and had lifestyle habits that were not in line with what we advocated.

Blue Cure was for me to share and amplify my story and message. Us men are inundated twenty-four-seven with unhealthy marketing and advertising messages everywhere: on social media, radio, print, television, at the movies, at arenas and stadiums, and so on. Everywhere we turn, there are advertisements enticing us to eat a high-sodium, nutrient-deficient, high-fat, and sugar-laden food product created by a food scientist. Worse is that male professional athletes influence our purchasing decisions for many unhealthy foods. This was part of the problem, and it intersected with our health, masculinity, and hardened stigma.

I was at dinner, catching up with friends I hadn't seen in a while. I told them I wanted their feedback for an idea I had for Men's Health Month, an observance not widely known or supported by hospitals and businesses, nor reported in the media.

My friends were a few margaritas deep in conversation. I jumped in, "Listen. Do you agree the phrase 'men's health' should be reframed to encourage younger men to pay attention to their health and take action?"

A few eyebrows lifted. I knew we were all there to kick back and relax, but I had to ask. What I was about to share with them had been on my mind.

"Sorry to be so serious, guys. I want to bounce this off you. Did you know that in America, more men than women die from heart disease, cancer, suicide, accidents, diabetes, and kidney disease? Men lead women in six of the top ten leading causes of death. You won't see these stats on the news during Men's Health Month. There won't be any media coverage during Men's Health Month."

"You wouldn't know that because of how 'men's health' issues are framed and marketed to us. It doesn't help there's a disproportionate amount of attention on women's health issues from the media, hospitals and cancer centers, and businesses with their cause-related marketing campaigns. Men barely get a fraction of it, and it's mostly wives and women who complain to me there isn't enough attention on men's health."

I had seen it and lived it for nine years.

"Are you getting ready for a media interview, Gabe?"

Laughs.

"I'm contemplating taking a drive for men's health. Literally a drive to raise awareness. I believe by sharing my story of early-stage prostate cancer and how it was tied to poor lifestyle habits passed down in my family, I can capture attention, reach younger men, and encourage action against obesity, heart disease, stroke, diabetes, and other chronic disease and mental health issues. I know others will relate to the story of my family and living with lifestyle-driven chronic disease that could have been prevented with annual checkups and proper lifestyle advice and encouragement. They all had faith in pills to get them healthy, but they got worse. My family's choices led to premature death and a poor quality of life. My choices led to early-stage prostate cancer. You following?"

A few nods.

"Poor mental health led to my stepdad dying by suicide when I was young, and my inability to properly cope led to unhealthy behaviors as I got older, which contributed to my poor health: overweight, high cholesterol, and early-stage prostate cancer. I want to share more of my mental health challenges and help end the shame men have in talking about it. There's a direct line that can be drawn to poor mental health and poor physical health."

I had seen numerous "men's health" campaigns over the years that mostly called attention to prostate and testicular cancers, and some also brought attention to mental health issues. Men's health needed to be reframed so men could view health issues more than what's exclusive to our anatomy, "To save lives, 'men's health' has to be reframed so that it's not focused mostly on testicular cancer, prostate cancer, low T, and hair loss."

I asked what they thought about me going on a men's health road tour around Texas. I would drive from Houston to Dallas, southwest to Austin, further south to San Antonio, out west to El Paso, and back.

"Each city I visit, I plan to highlight local men's health statistics like obesity, heart disease, lung cancer, and suicide and share information on prevention and local health resources that are free or subsidized. I hope to amplify the message by securing local media to encourage viewers to schedule a checkup and adopt healthy habits. I'll push the campaign through social media and a website specific to the campaign."

They paused, as if to wait for me to continue. "Sounds great, Gabe."

That wasn't really the reaction I wanted. I thought about it for a second and asked, "What if I drive from Houston to Los Angeles and back?"

Nods of approval. They continued their conversation.

"What if I drive from Houston to California, up the coast to Seattle, and back?"

Before they could react, "What if I drive from Houston, up the West Coast to Seattle, then from Seattle, hitting cities across America to New York City, down to Florida and back to Houston? I'll drive through twenty, thirty, forty cities around America to raise awareness of men's health issues!"

"You're crazy, Gabe! That's insane!"

I smiled, "Well, then, that's what I'm going to do!"

I began to put the idea into action. I planned the route I would drive, compiled a list of municipal and state health departments, and developed a new website that would provide visitors and media with national, state, and local men's health data and resources for the places I would visit. The campaign was last-minute and was a culmination of my listening daily to my dad's stubbornness about his health and thousands of guys I was talking to that weren't taking their health seriously, waiting till a diagnosis to act.

We didn't have sponsors to cover accommodations and expenses. This campaign would be on a shoestring budget. But my board members were encouraging and saw the upside. Their support made the campaign a reality. We discussed me scheduling the meetings with the pharmaceutical representatives the consultants had recommended. I rationalized that pharmaceutical companies generate billions in annual revenue and make contributions to cancer nonprofits. Couldn't they support some Blue Cure educational initiatives to encourage men—especially Hispanic and Black men with higher rates of overweight, obesity, chronic disease, and prostate cancer—to make simple lifestyle changes for better health and stave off disease? Would there be a catch? I would soon find out.

As I drove through cities and states, my plan was to post daily updates on my personal social media and Blue Cure's much larger platform. I would pitch media ahead of time to try to secure an interview and offer story suggestions for Men's Health Month with a call to action for their viewers. I believed local news reporters would bite, report on the campaign, and share the statistics I provided. I also suggested they interview a local doctor or male who was recovering from bypass surgery or a lung or prostate cancer survivor. Journalists are always looking for content that is newsworthy, relevant, and timely. I was giving them that, and it served the public. The local and national men's health data was alarming and supported my pitch that men are dying prematurely, are sick, and simple lifestyle changes can help stave off early death and lead to a higher quality of life. That was my one, two, three pitch to media, and I would tailor each pitch using local statistics and resources. This would be an opportunity to have journalists share more information about local health resources, free screenings wherever available, interview medical professionals, dietitians, men who survived heart attacks, stroke, and other illnesses. This was about reframing men's health, and I needed the media to help shape that narrative.

I reached out to the deputy editor of a major news distribution service. He had previously worked in television news, and I had known him for years. We had previously discussed the media coverage on men's health issues, which I would complain over and over is a fraction of the coverage women's health issues receive. He heard me say repeatedly that news organizations could do more and better by not framing the occasional "men's health" story exclusive to prostate or testicular cancer. There needed to be many more stories reported on the sky-high rates of males with obesity, heart disease, stroke, diabetes—chronic diseases that are mostly lifestyle-driven. The men in my family could have benefitted from more media stories. Also, there was the shame men had in discussing a prostate cancer diagnosis and overall health issues, and I believed just by having more stories on "men's health," men would begin to feel more comfortable and open to discussing and acting.

Media coverage showing health data on males, especially younger men, not consistently scheduling annual checkups and the continual increase in obesity and chronic diseases could serve as a wake-up call.

He acknowledged men's health issues deserved much more media attention. He encouraged me to have conversations with everyday men in communities around America. "Ask questions. Look for common threads. Go on a fact-finding mission," he said. "You have an incredible story, and you never know what you could learn through this experience and apply to your advocacy. What you'll be doing on the trip is newsworthy. You might get some media, but don't count on it. I'll be available for advice."

Before I left Houston, I met with Dr. Cohen to record a series of videos framing men's health as whole-body, and he advocated the need for sleep, love and support, exercise, stress management, avoiding environmental toxins, and encouraging a plant-centered diet. He refers to these points as the "Mix of Six" approach to reducing cancer and chronic disease and improving mental health. I could always count on Lorenzo being available when I needed him to record his expertise and encouraging words. It was the right video series to kick off the campaign.

> Fox 26 News Anchor, Rashi Vats: "H-town is the first stop on a 7,800-mile road trip to raise awareness for men's health issues. We have Gabe Canales here with the advocacy group Blue Cure to talk about the journey he's about to start later this morning. This is going to be a long journey happening in a few hours."

> Gabe Canales: "It's going to be worth it though."

> Rashi Vats: "Tell me about it."

> Gabe Canales: "According to the Cleveland Clinic, only three in five men get an annual checkup, and 60% of all men do not go to the doctor when they fear a serious medical condition. I know having run Blue Cure for over eight years that men don't like to talk about their health

issues. Men's health is mental health, men's health is heart health, its prostate health, its sexual health, its issues that men feel like they lose their masculinity when they talk about these issues, and they just have a fear of knowing. So, I want to destigmatize some of these issues and really get guys going to the doctor, getting an annual checkup and being more open about some of these issues. It's important, 3.5 times as many men commit suicide, and you've got other issues that men need to confront. And I want to help them get there."[48]

I hit the road with no guarantees in front of me. My fifty-five-pound Australian Shepherd, Sparky, was along for the long ride. I couldn't leave him. A month before, his older brother Lucky had passed away, and it hit me hard. Lucky was my first dog and had been there comforting me when I was diagnosed with prostate cancer. He sensed how sad I was and was always at my side when I was at the house.

I was driving into Austin and hadn't heard back from any of the Austin media outlets I had pitched a few days earlier. I went to a Starbucks downtown, where I met with the web designer volunteering her time and talent to develop and update the website used for the campaign. As a mother to a son and a wife, she believed in the message and the purpose of the trip and was more than happy to support the cause. That meant a lot. We walked a few blocks, where I held a sign over my head with the Texas State Capitol behind me as my backdrop. The sign read:

> 74% of persons who died in Austin
> by suicide (2013–2017) were males.
> –City of Austin.
> –Mental Health is Men's Health–
> Austin, Texas
> June is #MensHealthMonth[49]

Yes, on purpose, I wanted the first sign and statistic to be about suicide and mental health. This trip would be about pointing out statistics and stories that might bring discomfort. I couldn't worry about that. I needed to share what wasn't normally shared and discussed. Let the chips fall where they may.

I posted the photo holding the sign on all my and Blue Cure's social media accounts, reminding supporters and asking strangers to follow me on the journey around America to encourage men to commit to their health and take action. I also added men's health statistics and additional information for Austin on the campaign website. This would be the model I would use for each city I would visit: I would pitch media ahead of time, see if there was a doctor or subject matter expert I could meet with, post local statistics and available resources, identify a landmark in the city I could take a photo in front of holding a sign with a men's health statistic, post it to social media, engage men in conversation at cafes, restaurants, coffee shops, grocery stores, gas stations, hospitals—wherever I could. I would tell them what I was doing and ask if they would be open to talking about men's health.

I didn't hear back from any of the local Austin media I had pitched, and I was off on a short hour and a half drive to San Antonio, where I planned to meet with my father.

My sign for San Antonio would be in front of the Alamo. A stranger agreed to take my photo, and a small crowd of tourists gathered around to read what was on the sign I held.

78% of men in San Antonio / Bexar County
are overweight and obese.
City of San Antonio
Metropolitan Health District
San Antonio, Texas
June is #MensHealthMonth[50]

Seventy-eight percent! That is a jaw-dropping statistic. San Antonio is the largest Hispanic-majority city. My obese Hispanic father and other overweight and obese family members live in San Antonio and South Texas, and the root cause of their health issues is poor diet. It was mine. I was frustrated that my father's and family members' doctors never talked to them about their dietary habits. We live in an age of body-positive images that can do more harm than good. My family members never saw their weight as an issue. They were dealt a disservice by culture and their doctors. Many Hispanics in South Texas need to hear the truth, and this formerly overweight Hispanic gladly wanted to bring it to their attention.

As I positioned myself holding the sign, something bizarre happened. A police officer screamed at me and told me I can't take a photo in front of the Alamo holding that sign. He was obese. I asked the officer why. The stranger taking my photo handed back my phone, and the officer yelled, "Get out of here!"

"Why?"

I didn't get an answer.

"I have prostate cancer, and I'm raising awareness for men's health issues, and this is part of a campaign. Men in San Antonio are obese and need to lose weight to save themselves!"

"Get out of here!" he yelled.

I couldn't believe it. Did my sign trigger him? I was shocked, but I wasn't about to give up.

I walked down the street, and a few minutes later, I walked right back in front of the Alamo, just not as close as my original position. A photo would still capture the Alamo behind me. I asked another stranger to take my photo, and he started taking photos, guiding me to, "Move a little to the left, a few steps back, hold it above your head, hold it next to your waist."

As he was taking the photos, I heard shouting. I turned and saw the obese officer again, this time with two more obese officers, all slowly running towards me. The sight was incredible. I grabbed my camera phone from the stranger, thanked him, and sprinted to my car. When I got to my car, I laughed my ass off at how ridiculous the ordeal was. I checked my phone and saw the stranger had taken some good photos I could use, and I posted one of them.

I then visited my dad with the hope he would agree to be in a video of us having a conversation about his poor health, the unhealthy lifestyle habits of the men in our family, and the role machismo and pride played in not confronting health issues, leading to poor health and premature death.

The next day, my father and I went through a McDonald's drive-through and ordered salads. My father eats lots of fast food burgers, and his reasons are they're "cheap, quick, and satisfying." I wanted to show my dad you can also order a healthy food item at McDonald's. He agreed to order a salad as a favor to me. Mine was a salad with extra vegetables and no meat; his was a bacon ranch chicken salad. He didn't even know they sold salads but told me later the salad was "so-so" and didn't compare to a burger.

We recorded a video in the front seat of his car, and he said heart disease, diabetes, and stroke were passed down in the family. At first, he didn't attribute his poor health to poor dietary habits, but he acknowledged they all pretty much ate the same. It's what they knew. They never believed the way they ate was bad for their health. But it was. It was a revealing and honest conversation between us. We had never had a conversation like that, and I was grateful he allowed me to record and share it. I had never shared a private conversation before, nor had I openly shared my father's health challenges and that of the men in my family. After I posted that video, I received quite a few responses from people who could relate, and they desperately wanted to break the pattern. Being open and vulnerable was connecting with others.

Before I left town, I shot a video with representatives of Salud America! at UT Health San Antonio, "a national Latino-focused organization that creates culturally relevant and research-based stories, videos, and tools to inspire people to start and support healthy changes." Since I started my advocacy in 2010, I've worked to highlight health disparities and stigma among men in the Hispanic community. Just by sharing my story, I've had numerous Hispanic men reach out to engage me about their health issues or that of a family member. Years earlier, I had launched campaigns for Blue Cure en Español to confront linguistic and cultural barriers. It's obviously personal to me because of my family.

Also, early on in my conversations with Dr. Rod Paige, I was mindful of prostate cancer incidence and death amongst African American males. It's why during my trip, I sought out prostate cancer survivor and African American Freddie Muse, founder of The Men's Cancer Network Inc. in Los Angeles. During my visit to Cleveland, I met with African American

Charles Modlin, MD, at the Cleveland Clinic. Dr. Modlin is a renowned kidney transplant surgeon and urologist, and he is the founder of Cleveland Clinic's Minority Men's Health Center and Health Fair. I recorded a series of videos with both men during my visits to Los Angeles and Cleveland, discussing racial health disparities and encouraging men of color to be proactive and make lifestyle changes.

Hispanics and Blacks have higher rates of obesity, chronic disease, and cancers. It was important for me to raise these issues and awareness of minority mental health as part of the campaign. Too much stigma and shame exist among Black and Hispanic men to confront health issues. I wanted to chip away at those issues.

The trip around America is a book in and of itself, but of the more than forty cities I visited, these are a sampling of the places I visited across America with a top-line statistic on the signs I held up:

> At the Santa Monica Pier in California, the sign I held read: "92% of early syphilis cases in Los Angeles County are males." Men's Health is Sexual Health.[51]

> In White Sands, New Mexico: "Lung cancer is the #1 cause of cancer death in New Mexican Men and 90% of lung cancer cases are attributable to cigarette smoking."[52]

> In front of the Washington State Capitol in Olympia, Washington: "Prostate Cancer is the most commonly diagnosed cancer among men in Washington State, and Lung Cancer is the leading cause of death among males."[53]

> In front of Seattle's Space Needle, I held a sign that pointed to the high rates of male suicide in King County.[54]

> In front of the Utah State Capitol in Salt Lake City: "Prostate cancer is the most commonly diagnosed male cancer in men in Utah."[55]

In Notre Dame, Indiana: "23.5% of Indiana males reported they currently smoke every day or some days, and 73% of Indiana males are overweight and obese."[56]

In front of the Idaho State Capitol in Des Moines, the sign read that 72% of Iowa males were overweight and obese.[57]

In the middle of New York City's Times Square: "Lung Cancer is the leading cause of death for New York males and 68.4% of males are overweight and obese."[58]

In front of the National Cancer Instituter in Bethesda, Maryland: "1 in 3 men will develop cancer in his lifetime."[59]

In front of the Washington Monument in Washington, DC: "1 in 4 male deaths in America are from heart disease."[60]

In front of the Centers for Disease Control and Prevention in Atlanta, Georgia: "73.7% of adult males in America are overweight and obese, with annual estimated costs ranging from $147 billion to $210 billion."[61]

In front of the Alabama State Capitol in Montgomery: "72% of Alabama males are overweight and obese."[62]

In front of the Biloxi Lighthouse landmark in Biloxi, Mississippi: "74.3% of males are overweight and obese."[63]

These are some of the people I met with and shared recordings about:

In Sausalito, California, I met with Dr. Dean Ornish, and we recorded a series of videos discussing mental health, depression, and suicide. Dr. Ornish framed "men's health" as whole body—to have a healthy heart, mind, erections, and stave off disease. He showed me an extended preview of the James Cameron film, *The Game Changers*, which emphasized men eating plant-based for prevention and athleticism. I was more than happy to promote this film during the campaign.

In Portland, I met with Dr. Tomasz Beer at the Oregon Health & Science University's Knight Cancer Institute. Dr. Beer leads the Prostate Cancer Research Program. We discussed the basics of prostate cancer and PSA testing.

In New York City, I recorded videos with urologist Dr. Ketan Badani, the vice chairman of urology and robotic operations at Mount Sinai Health System. We discussed the age a man should be screened for prostate cancer, the accuracy of PSA testing, genomic and genetic testing, and other issues around prostate cancer.

In Salt Lake City, Utah, I visited with urologist Alexander Pastuszak of Utah Men's Health. Dr. Pastuszak provided a series of videos for the campaign on causes and medications for erectile dysfunction and the mental and sexual side effects of hair loss medications.

I met with Joseph Gonzales in Park City, Utah. Joseph was the former director of nutrition for Blue Cure. We recorded a video on mental health, and he opened about his struggles with addiction. He had never been public about that, but he wanted to share his struggles to help end the stigma around men talking about addiction and mental health.

In Seattle, I recorded videos with Colby Wallace, a father who was posting motivational signs in his neighborhood that read "Don't Give Up" and "You Are Enough" to combat a spike in local teen suicides. He had received local and national media attention, and I wanted to meet

him and discuss how men feel shame when confronting
our mental health challenges and need to seek out help.

Early in the campaign, a seasoned, experienced Hollywood publicist reached out and asked how it was going. She had been following it on social media. I shared the challenges I was experiencing not getting the coverage I expected. She offered to help at no charge. I was incredibly grateful. She began to send press releases ahead of time to media outlets in the cities I would soon visit. Each press release was tailored with men's health statistics for that city and state, but she began to encounter what I knew all too well. She would speak to assignments editors and reporters and would receive feedback there wasn't any interest in covering men's health issues. They just didn't have the time to do it, but generally, there wasn't any interest. Some would say they had done a story on prostate cancer earlier in the year. She was beside herself at the responses. She didn't understand why they didn't see the newsworthiness. Neither did I, but I was on the inside looking out, and hearing her frustration was what I had experienced and seen for years.

I did have television interviews in Eugene, Seattle, Charlotte, Cleveland, and Raleigh—far less than what I expected—and I expressed my frustration with the deputy editor at the news-gathering organization I had spoken with as I began the trip. I shared the feedback from the publicist helping me. She was running into a wall. It was what he and I had previously discussed. That's when the deputy editor asked about his organization doing a story on my road trip. He said it deserved to be reported. He said it would be widely distributed, on television stations across America, reaching tens of millions of viewers. I was elated. This was huge.

It was undeniable. Everywhere I looked, almost every guy I had engaged in a conversation—whether in the middle of the country at a gas station, at a cafe in a suburban community, at a coffee shop in an urban area—was overweight and obese. It's one thing to read the national and local statistics; it's another when you see it up close, seemingly everywhere.

It was also challenging to find healthy options during my 8,867 miles of travels. Fast food chains dotted the interstate highways, and almost all gas stations and rest stops offered only high-sugar drinks and ultra-processed junk foods. A few times, I would find a banana or an apple for sale at a gas station. Not surprisingly, customers checking out were mostly overweight and obese, holding bottles of soda, chips, and a candy bar, asking the attendant for a pack of cigarettes. (Again, the number one cause of cancer death for men was 90 percent attributable to cigarette smoking.)[64]

I did have quite a few conversations with men in their twenties to late seventies. I would randomly strike up conversations wherever I could and tell strangers I was living with prostate cancer and driving across America to raise awareness of men's health issues. I would ask if they had a few minutes to chat. Some would instantly say no and just walk away; others gave me a few minutes. Off the top and not surprisingly, most men I spoke with were overweight, many were obese, most didn't schedule an annual checkup, and most told me when they had visited a doctor, their diet and lifestyle had never been asked about nor discussed. One hundred percent of the men I spoke with said they could never eat a plant-based diet. (I had to explain what that was to most of them.) Many said they rarely ate fruits and vegetables. Some of the older men I met expressed more of a desire to feel better and live longer. I asked every man I spoke with what the number one killer of men was. Some guessed prostate cancer, others said cancer, a few said heart disease, and others just wouldn't say. Most men I spoke with weren't getting screened for prostate cancer or discussing screenings with a physician. When I asked what "men's health" meant to them, many said erections or erectile dysfunction, some said prostates, some said exercising, and some didn't know what to say.

I was exhausted and mentally spent when I completed the trip, which ended up being 8,867 miles. I was filled with mixed emotions. So much about this seven-week road trip was disheartening, but clarity would ensue.

"I'm sorry, Gabe. My boss killed it."

I laugh.

Silence.

"Wait, are you serious?

"Yes, I'm sorry."

"I don't understand. You're the boss!"

"I have a boss."

"Last week, you sent a photojournalist to Houston to take photos of me running at Memorial Park. He showed me the completed story on his phone that would soon be available to TV stations. It was a strong piece."

"He shouldn't have done that, Gabe."

"As I was driving through Georgia, you called telling me to drive two states back to Charlotte, for an on-camera interview with one of your reporters. The other day, you had me interview on the phone with two reporters for the print piece. Both TV and print pieces are dead? How?"

I was incensed. Desperately trying to make a case for him to reverse what he had just told me.

Months earlier, halfway into my drive around America for men's health, the deputy editor at the news-gathering and distribution service I had reached to for advice informed me that he was interested in covering my road trip and would assign a journalist to meet me. It was newsworthy. This was a huge confidence booster. The story would include an on-camera interview, and the "package" would be distributed to TV stations across the country. The exposure would be huge, reaching tens of millions of Americans, probably more than that. As the date approached for the release of the story, the deputy editor contacted me, saying they would also like to interview me for a piece to be distributed for print to newspapers across America.

"Gabe, I am angry too! This story deserves to be told. Do you think I would have allocated resources and had a reporter meet you in person for an on-camera segment, had a photographer meet you in Houston for a photo shoot, and had a journalist speak with you by phone if I didn't believe this would happen?"

"After I interviewed with your journalist in North Carolina, I stopped pitching local news stations the rest of the road trip! You said a nicely produced package would be available to the stations I would be pitching."

"I do believe it's a story, and I'm sorry. I'm angry at my bosses for doing this. Look, Gabe. I wanted this for you. I know you've worked so hard, and you're very passionate. The issues you're working on deserve media attention. We need more reporting on men's health issues. But don't look at this as a failure. For all you know, you could write a book about all this. You should write a book."

In 2012, a few years after I started Blue Cure, I was visiting my parents for dinner, and while I was in the kitchen peeking at the food my mother was preparing, she unexpectedly grabbed a roll of my stomach fat over my shirt.

"What are you doing, Mom?!"

"Look at this! You have got to get this under control. You started Blue Cure to help men by promoting healthy habits and prevention. Look at you!"

I was shocked.

"Practice what you preach!"

I turned to my stepdad, looking for his help, "Who does that? Who says that?"

I was angry. "I look great! I'm just a big guy. No one else has told me I'm fat."

"Well, I'm your mother, and I'm worried about your health. Your doctor told you what you eat could affect the growth of your prostate cancer, and your father's side of the family has lots of heart problems, and they're all overweight!"

I was offended, and I left.

That night, before getting in the shower, I stared at my body in the mirror.

I grabbed my stomach. Yeah, there was a roll, and it was fat. It wasn't muscle.

My anger turned to sadness.

I had slipped into old habits, convincing myself each time I had snuck in a fast food meal here and there or alcohol, "it's just this time" and "it's in moderation."

I've said it before, and I'll say it again: I've come to believe "moderation" is an enabling word. Yeah, for someone already in great shape or for someone without early-stage prostate cancer, heart disease or diabetes, 'moderation' is okay. But for me, it wasn't. It was permission to continue to eat unhealthily.

My daily meetings with the mirror staring at my reflection while brushing my teeth and getting ready had been deceitful. I didn't think I looked overweight, but photos show I had gained weight. I had also been leaving my shirts tucked out.

We see what we want to see, and we don't see what we don't want to see.

I was so shaken by my mother's words that the next week I saw a nutritionist, and the calipers told the truth. My body fat percentage had increased sharply.

As I sat across from the nutritionist, he asked me, "You believe what you eat can lead to progression of your prostate cancer, right? That's what your doctor told you, and you believe this?"

"I do."

"You really believe that?"

"I do."

"If you believe that, why aren't your actions reflecting it? Your measurements reveal your actions and tell a story of unhealthy actions."

That stung.

We discussed triggers, my environment, and how to navigate these challenges.

I could have stayed angry about the way my mother approached my weight, but the fact that she did it had an effect that led me to act and see a nutritionist, really take stock and reflect on my habits and triggers, and make changes.

I needed to hear her jolting words. My mom was right. You may disagree with how she did it, but I look back at that incident as critical in my journey to better health.

I deeply believe a lot of men need to have someone speak truth about their weight.

Why is this an issue?

According to the CDC:

> "People who have obesity, compared to those with a normal or healthy weight, are at increased risk for many

serious diseases and health conditions, including the following:[65]

- All-causes of death (mortality)
- High blood pressure (Hypertension)
- High LDL cholesterol, low HDL cholesterol, or high levels of triglycerides (Dyslipidemia)
- Type 2 diabetes
- Coronary heart disease
- Stroke
- Gallbladder disease
- Osteoarthritis (a breakdown of cartilage and bone within a joint)
- Sleep apnea and breathing problems
- Many types of cancer
- Low quality of life
- Mental illness such as clinical depression, anxiety, and other mental disorders
- Body pain and difficulty with physical functioning"

The CDC also states:[66]

"Being overweight or having obesity increases your risk of getting cancer. You may be surprised to learn that being overweight or having obesity are linked with a higher risk of getting 13 types of cancer. These cancers make up 40% of all cancers diagnosed in the United States each year."

The American Institute for Cancer Research states:[67]

- There is strong evidence that being overweight or obese increases the risk of advanced prostate cancer.
- Obesity influences the levels of a number of hormones and growth factors. Insulin and leptin are elevated in people with obesity and can promote the growth of cancer cells.

- Sex steroid hormones, including estrogen, androgen, and progesterone, are likely to play a role in obesity and cancer. In men, obesity is related to lower serum testosterone levels, which in turn may be associated with enhanced risk of or adverse outcome in advanced prostate cancer.
- Obesity is characterized by a low-grade chronic inflammatory state. Such chronic inflammation can promote cancer development.

In 2010, it was eye-opening when my urologist told me my lifestyle habits contributed to my prostate cancer. But it gave me hope and a sense of empowerment when he said going forward that my weight and lifestyle habits could slow or reverse the progression of my early-stage disease.

I also felt more empowered knowing those lifestyle changes I was making to lose weight could also prevent me from getting heart disease, stroke, and diabetes—conditions that afflicted members of my family.

I worked to change my habits, and in the beginning, the pendulum swung way to the other side of plant-based eating and healthy lifestyle habits. But triggers arose, I stumbled, and I got complacent.

I recognized when I was slipping but failed to acknowledge the gradual changes in my appearance.

As I continued to grow in my knowledge on the harms of overweight and obesity and the health benefits of lifestyle habits and consuming specific food groups, it became harder for me to succumb to triggers.

Each time, I consciously thought of the consequences: mentally, physically, and medically.

I recognize the power and influence of media, culture, and "body-positivity" messaging. I don't believe in shaming (though everyone can feel shame differently). However, I believe that fear has taken hold in discussing bodyweight: a fear of offending. I have spoken with countless overweight individuals who advocate self-acceptance for overweight and obesity. My concern is self-acceptance is leading to chronic disease and cancer and not scheduling a visit to the physician for an annual checkup.

I've heard, "You don't think overweight people know they're overweight?"

No, I don't believe all overweight people believe they're overweight.

If media and culture promote self-acceptance for all body sizes, when would a man think he is overweight—or at an unhealthy weight? Overweight becomes "normal," but "normal" isn't healthy.

Walk into the men's section of the department store, and you'll see mannequins are larger and clothing sizes have increased. Our culture celebrates "dad bods," which further promotes unhealthy behavior.

Overweight and obesity—I've lived it. I've gut-wrenchingly experienced it with my family members, and I won't shy away from speaking the truth. I can't help it when others are offended.

CHAPTER SIXTEEN

CONCLUSION—MEN'S HEALTH: THE HEART OF THE PROBLEM

I get asked many times about the right age to get a PSA test for prostate cancer. I always ask if they get annual checkups and if they've discussed with their physician whether they should be screened for prostate cancer. The response is usually, "It's been a few years since I've been to the doctor for a checkup."

I can't tell you how common a response that is. Most of the men I speak with haven't gotten an annual checkup in years, and if they did, they don't remember much about it. They aren't able to give me basic numbers like their cholesterol and blood pressure. I often hear, "But I'm healthy!" (I also thought I was "healthy" when I learned I had high cholesterol, was overweight, had high body fat, and low testosterone.) And let's be honest, most men are not healthy when data shows 73.7 percent of adult men in America are overweight and have obesity.[68]

I've learned a lot in my journey in the search for answers on how to treat my prostate cancer. I learned the role of lifestyle quality and how it played in my diagnosis. I took stock of decades of poor lifestyle habits and those of my family members who struggled for years with health problems and died prematurely of chronic diseases. A common thread I recognized was that all my family members, including myself, with poor health, lived decades with harmful dietary and lifestyle habits, naively not understanding the gravity and consequences of our everyday choices. We were each dealing with being overweight and obesity, high cholesterol, high blood pressure, diabetes, stroke, heart attack, aneurysm, and in my case, early-stage prostate cancer.

To my family members, "health care" was reactive and included handfuls of prescription pills to treat only the symptoms. My father is currently taking sixteen prescription pills every day. He and my other family members never received counseling on lifestyle and dietary interventions to improve and reverse their conditions and to stave off an early death.

Learning at age thirty-five that I had slow-growing early-stage prostate cancer was a blessing. It was my wake-up call. It saved me. I was heading down the same miserable path I helplessly witnessed members of my family head down. I didn't have the knowledge I now possess. If I did, I would have spoken up and encouraged change sooner. That's the thing about having knowledge—I can positively make a difference in others' lives. I feel compelled to share it.

I knew I didn't want to suffer, like my family, with poor health that affected their quality of life and led to an early death. I can still see my uncle eating his fast food burger, breathing heavily, moving slowly, just weeks before his passing from a major heart attack; my always-tired grandmother eating a plateful of fried chicken wings and tamales shortly before her passing; and my father recovering from a stroke, dealing with high blood pressure, eating barbecue, and using a cane to get around. My family's dietary habits down the ancestry line served as my motivation to seek alternative solutions to improve my health.

As I learned, I realized I had more control over my health than I thought possible. I was empowered. I grew up hearing, "Heart attacks and diabetes run in the family." The truth is poor habits ran in my family. Chronic diseases were not my predetermined fate. My knowledge and choices were my power. With that came responsibility and accountability.

My diagnosis had me examine if other men had a similar experience regarding their health. I asked questions and began to recognize how men view health issues that affect us most, like heart disease, obesity, lung cancer, mental health, and suicide. My marketing and public relations background spurred me to analyze how key influencers of men—media, sports, and celebrity—add to the stigma we have in addressing our health issues, contributing to why we are so slow to act.

Throughout my advocacy and travels around America, I've met tens of thousands of men of all ages, from all walks of life. I've met prostate cancer survivors, caretakers, and men with various chronic diseases. I've asked about their lifestyle and dietary habits, cultural norms, what led to their diagnosis, and whether they were getting annual checkups. I've had many revealing conversations with men opening up and sharing things they hadn't before. I've learned from them. I'm honored and grateful to have been confided in and trusted.

I've also had discussions and heard perspectives from physicians, urologists, oncologists, cancer researchers, cardiologists, lifestyle medicine experts, dietitians, public health department representatives, elected leaders, pharmaceutical representatives, professional athletes, and journalists. There's wide agreement that men's health doesn't get enough attention, and that prevention isn't widely taught, advocated, and promoted. It's also not where the money is.

When I shared I had prostate cancer with a few friends and acquaintances, I began to realize how rare my diagnosis was. I learned all my friends in their twenties to forties had never been checked for prostate cancer. Most of them didn't know a thing about their prostate. It makes sense when you consider the median age of diagnosis for prostate cancer is sixty-seven, the median age of death is eighty, and all the marketing and awareness campaigns use imagery of much older men with white hair.

In those first few years, outside of a few medical conferences where I spoke, I was speaking to audiences of younger men, college-age to young professionals. Occasionally, I was asked to speak to high school athletes. Men that age rarely, if ever, receive education about prostate cancer—and certainly not from someone at my younger age who was living with it. When I spoke to men ages twenty to forty, I was able to see their reactions, and I gained a unique insight from their feedback that was valuable in shaping my perspective. I would hear about a father or grandfather who was a prostate cancer survivor, but the questions would be asked whether they should get screened for prostate cancer. The controversial guidelines for prostate cancer screenings were to discuss with your doctor at age fifty-five and older. Though younger men found my story interesting, how could my story motivate them to act now? Talking about "prostate cancer" wasn't getting younger men to act. Some participated in fundraisers for prostate cancer research, but besides raising funds, how could I encourage them to become proactive with their health care?

When I've asked men, "What is men's health?" the overwhelming responses are "erectile dysfunction, low testosterone, and balding." This is how a lot (most) men I've had discussions with over ten-plus years define "men's health," and it's the result of tens of millions of drug company marketing and advertising dollars.

My case made me wonder how many men in their thirties with no family history of prostate cancer but who are overweight, stressed, and consuming inflammatory foods are walking around with no idea they have early-stage prostate cancer?

I realized that to get through to more men and have a greater impact when sharing my story, I had to reframe the phrase "men's health." To move the needle and save lives, I had to share more of my family's story, which, I would learn, is a story similar in many American families.

I began to share startling statistics that more younger men were able to relate to. Most were surprised to learn that over 70 percent of males in America are overweight and obese. More were surprised to learn that in America, over half of all men twenty years of age and older have cardiovascular disease. Half of all men twenty years of age and older have high blood pressure. High blood pressure can lead to heart attack, stroke, and erectile dysfunction. Mention boners, and you have their attention.

What could prompt men to act earlier? I thought of what I believed had the greatest return on investment—and the greatest reward for optimal health and prevention. It was simple. It's at the center of each of us.

The key to prostate health and men's health starts with our heart.

My prostate cancer journey led me to my heart. The disease journey of my family led me to the heart.

Why start with the heart? Heart disease is our number one killer. Heart disease kills eleven times more men annually than prostate cancer. I learned early on in my research that there was a connection and that heart health was the foundation to optimal health. The good news, according to the CDC, is at least 80 percent of heart disease is preventable with diet and lifestyle changes. This is low-hanging fruit. Hundreds of thousands of lives could be saved by making different lifestyle choices. The ripple effect would be a massive tidal wave, saving trillions in health-care costs.

If men placed a greater focus on heart health starting at a younger age, we would have fewer cases of prostate cancer, obesity, high blood pressure, lung cancer, heart disease, diabetes, stroke, erectile dysfunction, and suicide.

In 2011, I watched Dr. Manny Alvarez say on Fox News, "A diet that's good for your prostate is also good for your heart."[69]

I thought of his words all that day. They resonated with me and confirmed what I was learning. I believed it, but I framed it differently based on what I was learning, "A diet that's good for your heart is also good for your lungs, prostate, brain, kidneys, liver, sexual health, erections, and overall health."

How is that?

Early in my journey, after my meeting with Dr. Katz, I became immersed in research on diet, lifestyle, and cancer. I read Dean Ornish's research papers on "Intensive Lifestyle Changes for Reversal of Coronary Heart Disease" and "Intensive Lifestyle Changes May Affect the Progression of Prostate Cancer." Those were game-changers that convinced me of a connection between lifestyle and chronic disease and cancer.

That year, Dr. Ornish's diet was rated "The #1 Best Heart Healthy Diet" by *U.S. News & World Report*, and the panel of nutrition experts continue to rate the Ornish Diet number one for the tenth year, from 2011 to 2021.[70]

It is this heart-healthy, anti-inflammatory diet that I adopted, along with other crucial lifestyle changes, including a strong emphasis on mental health. Dr. Ornish's research shows that we can reverse coronary heart disease, type two diabetes, early-stage prostate cancer, high blood pressure, elevated cholesterol levels, and obesity.

These health issues affect many men, and they don't have to.

Dr. Ornish says the reason that these lifestyle changes can reverse the progression of so many different chronic diseases is that they are different manifestations of the same underlying biological mechanisms:

chronic inflammation, chronic sympathetic nervous system stimulation, microbiome and TMAO, oxidative stress, apoptosis, gene expression, telomeres, and the immune system.

I made these dietary and lifestyle changes believing they would slow and reverse the progression of my early-stage prostate cancer—AND I believed these changes would prevent me from suffering from coronary heart disease like my grandmother, uncle, and cousins; diabetes like my uncle; high blood pressure and an aneurysm like my grandpa and aunt; high cholesterol and a stroke like my dad; and high cholesterol like my mom.

What has been the effect of the dietary and lifestyle changes I adopted? I lost thirty-five pounds, and my body fat percent decreased. My elevated cholesterol went down drastically, and my blood pressure is normal. After decades of using prescription shampoos and topical medications for seborrheic dermatitis (a chronic inflammatory disorder), the crusty breakouts on my scalp, hairline, and around my nose stopped. My skin is clear. My PSA is lower than it was in 2011, and a repeat biopsy didn't find evidence of low-grade prostate cancer. My erections are better and firmer. I sleep better. My high-meat, low-fiber diet before my diagnosis gave me a bowel movement once a day with god-awful constipation and hemorrhoids. Eating high-fiber, plant-based whole foods, I'm never constipated, I don't have hemorrhoids, I never feel bloated, and I have bowel movements four or five times a day. My energy has increased.

Having optimal health for a strong immune system and prevention includes eating lots of high-fiber, nutrient-rich plants, exercising daily, managing stress by sharing more, journaling, seeing a therapist, spending as much time as possible in nature, getting plenty of sleep, and scheduling an annual checkup.

I can't stress enough the importance of annual checkups to have accountability, to stay on top of your weight, cholesterol, and blood pressure, and to discuss your family medical history of diseases and cancer. This is your time to be open, share, and ask questions with your physician.

If you have a family history of prostate cancer, have a conversation with your physician about a PSA test. If you have lived decades with unhealthy habits like I did, you could have early-stage prostate cancer. I do believe there are hundreds of thousands of men in their thirties walking around with early-stage prostate cancer and have no clue. Despite not having a family history of prostate cancer, if you spent years with poor lifestyle habits (poor sleep, not managing stress, smoking, excessive drinking) and a highly inflammatory diet, ask for a PSA test. Just know that strenuous activities like weightlifting, riding a bike, horseback riding, and sex will affect the results of your PSA. You should abstain from sex for two or three days, though some doctors I've talked to recommend abstaining for a week.

The results of your PSA test could lead to a referral to a urologist. Many prostate cancers are localized, and the key to catching prostate cancers at their earliest, most treatable and curable stage is to be consistent with annual checkups and have a discussion with your physician about getting checked for prostate cancer.

Unfortunately, because many men don't get annual checkups, they will put off visiting their primary care physician, and some will only get checked when they have symptoms indicating a more aggressive prostate cancer. You don't want prostate cancer to spread outside your prostate. That's a different ball game. Therefore, it's important to start annual checkups at a younger age.

These simple actions can save your life and improve your health:

1. Adopt a heart-healthy, high-fiber diet and lifestyle.
2. Get an annual checkup.
3. Avoid toxins and questionable chemicals as much as realistically possible.

I'm convinced that the foundation of men's health is heart health. This is my message for ALL MEN. It's a simple message. If you're good to your heart (eat plants, don't smoke, exercise, manage stress, etc.), your prostate and all other body parts will be good to you.

We often view our health issues as disparate, but they're all interconnected. We must look at the WHOLE.

Encouraging men starting at a younger age to get their annual physical is also an opportunity for openness in discussing sexual health and sexually transmitted infections, which are on the rise. There is no shame in asking questions and discussing these issues with your physician, and we must continue to encourage it to end the stigma.

Please, now, schedule an annual physical with your primary care physician.

COVID-19 brought to the forefront the consequences of America not confronting our obesity epidemic, our reactive health-care system, and our severe lack of focus on prevention. Despite the belief that America has the best health care in the world, we led, throughout the pandemic, in COVID-19 deaths. Factor in 73 percent of American adults are overweight or obese, six in ten adults in the US have a chronic disease, and four in ten adults have two or more. According to the CDC, 78 percent of COVID-19 patients hospitalized in the US were overweight or obese. Unfortunately, from the beginning and throughout the pandemic, our public health officials, elected leaders, and media gave almost no attention to the fact that unhealthy lifestyles played a major role in hospitalizations and deaths.[71]

We can't expect our leaders to save us. They won't. We each have a responsibility to our health.

I'm continuing to advocate for more attention targeting men and resources for men.

Collectively, we can bring about change.

Join me (follow on my socials) to call on:

1. Hospitals and cancer centers to target men with preventive messages (annual checkups and screenings) in their community outreach and marketing.
2. Local and national media, especially sports media, to package more stories and features of men and targeting men during February's American Heart Month, Cancer Prevention Month, September's National Prostate Cancer Month, Suicide Prevention Month, November's Lung Cancer Awareness Month, Diabetes Awareness Month and other observance months.
3. Local, state, and national government health departments and websites to allocate more funding, health information, and resources for men. When I traveled 8,867 miles around America

on the Blue Cure Men's Health Road Tour, I saw many local, state, and federal government and health department websites with a lot of information for women but not much for men. Many had no information for men. Community public health campaigns targeting men are also important to move the needle.

4. For the federal government's Department of Health and Human Services to establish an Office on Men's Health (OMH). In 1991, the Department of Health and Human Services established an Office on Women's Health (OWH) with ten women's health coordinators across the United States. The OWH functions to improve the health and well-being of U.S. women and girls.[72]

Thirty years later, still there is not an Office on Men's Health, and that's unacceptable. The life expectancy for males in America is six years shorter than women, and men lead women in six out of the top ten leading causes of death.

Change starts with you. Believe it! You have the power. Small changes lead to bigger changes and better health.

I will be encouraging you along the way in your journey to a healthier YOU!

ENDNOTES

Chapter One

[1] National Cancer Institute, "Treatment Choices for Men With Early-Stage Prostate Cancer," NIH Publication, January 2011, No. 11-4659, Page 3, https://www.cancer.gov/publications/patient-education/prostate-cancer-treatment-choices.pdf.

[2] American Cancer Society medical and editorial content team, "Prostate Cancer Risk Factors: Age," American Cancer Society, last modified June 9, 2020, https://www.cancer.org/cancer/prostate-cancer/causes-risks-prevention/risk-factors.html#:~:text=Prostate%20cancer%20is%20rare%20in,in%20men%20older%20than%2065.

[3] World Cancer Research Fund, "Prostate Cancer," American Institute for Cancer Research, https://www.wcrf.org/dietandcancer/prostate-cancer/.

[4] National Cancer Institute, "Cancer Stat Facts: Prostate Cancer," National Cancer Institute, last modified 2021, https://seer.cancer.gov/statfacts/html/prost.html.

[5] National Cancer Institute, "Cancer Stat Facts: Prostate Cancer," National Cancer Institute, last modified 2021, https://seer.cancer.gov/statfacts/html/prost.html.

[6] American Cancer Society medical and editorial content team, "Prostate Cancer Risk Factors: Family History," American Cancer Society, last modified June 9, 2020, https://www.cancer.org/cancer/prostate-cancer/causes-risks-prevention/risk-factors.html.

7   "Why Knowing Your Inherited Risk of Prostate Cancer Is Important," Cleveland Clinic, April 17, 2019, https://health.clevelandclinic.org/why-knowing-your-inherited-risk-of-prostate-cancer-is-important/.

8   American Cancer Society medical and editorial content team, "Prostate Cancer Risk Factors: Family history," American Cancer Society, last modified June 9, 2020, https://www.cancer.org/cancer/prostate-cancer/causes-risks-prevention/risk-factors.html.

9   American Cancer Society medical and editorial content team, "What Causes Prostate Cancer?: Acquired gene mutations," American Cancer Society, last modified August 1, 2019, https://www.cancer.org/cancer/prostate-cancer/causes-risks-prevention/what-causes.html.

10 "Who Is At Risk for Prostate Cancer?: African-American Men," CDC, last modified August 23, 2021, https://www.cdc.gov/cancer/prostate/basic_info/risk_factors.htm.

11 American Cancer Society, "PROSTATE CANCER FACTS & FIGURES IN BRIEF," American Cancer Society, last modified March 1, 2021, https://www.cancer.org/research/acs-research-highlights/prostate-cancer-research-highlights.html.

12 American Cancer Society, "Cancer Facts & Figures, Special Section: Prostate Cancer, How Many Cases and Deaths Are Estimated to Occur in 2010?" American Cancer Society, 2010,https://www.cancer.org/content/dam/cancer-org/research/cancer-facts-and-statistics/annual-cancer-facts-and-figures/2010/cancer-facts-and-figures-special-section-2010.pdf.

13 American Cancer Society, "PROSTATE CANCER FACTS & FIGURES IN BRIEF," American Cancer Society, last modified March 1, 2021, https://www.cancer.org/research/acs-research-highlights/prostate-cancer-research-highlights.html.

14 American Cancer Society, "PROSTATE CANCER FACTS & FIGURES IN BRIEF," American Cancer Society, last modified March 1, 2021, https://www.cancer.org/research/acs-research-highlights/prostate-cancer-research-highlights.html.

15 American Cancer Society, "PROSTATE CANCER FACTS & FIGURES IN BRIEF," American Cancer Society, last modified March 1, 2021,

https://www.cancer.org/research/acs-research-highlights/prostate-cancer-research-highlights.html.

16 National Cancer Institute, "Cancer Stat Facts: Prostate Cancer," National Cancer Institute, last modified 2021, https://seer.cancer.gov/statfacts/html/prost.html.

17 National Cancer Institute, "Cancer Stat Facts: Prostate Cancer," National Cancer Institute, last modified 2021, https://seer.cancer.gov/statfacts/html/prost.html.

18 National Cancer Institute, "Cancer Stat Facts: Prostate Cancer," National Cancer Institute, last modified 2021, https://seer.cancer.gov/statfacts/html/prost.html.

19 Email from Rachel Darwin, Public Relations Manager, National Comprehensive Cancer Network® (NCCN®).

20 American Cancer Society medical and editorial content team, "American Cancer Society Recommendations for Prostate Cancer Early Detection," American Cancer Society, last modified April 23, 2021, https://www.cancer.org/cancer/prostate-cancer/detection-diagnosis-staging/acs-recommendations.html.

21 "Final Recommendation Statement," U.S. Preventive Services Task Force, https://uspreventiveservicestaskforce.org/uspstf/announcements/final-recommendation-statement-screening-prostate-cancer.

22 "Prostate Cancer: Screening," U.S. Preventative Services Task Force, May 8, 2018, https://www.uspreventiveservicestaskforce.org/uspstf/recommendation/prostate-cancer-screening; "Final Recommendation Statement," U.S. Preventive Services Task Force, https://uspreventiveservicestaskforce.org/uspstf/announcements/final-recommendation-statement-screening-prostate-cancer.

23 Carter HB, Albertsen PC, and Barry MJ, "Early detection of prostate cancer," AUA Guideline, The Journal of Urology 190, no. 419 (last modified 2018), https://www.auanet.org/guidelines/guidelines/prostate-cancer-early-detection-guideline.

Chapter Two

24 "Isotretinoin Capsule Information," U.S. Food and Drug Administration, last modified October 12, 2021, https://www.fda.gov/drugs/postmarket-drug-safety-information-patients-and-providers/isotretinoin-capsule-information; Kristin Compton, "Accutane Side Effects," drugwatch, last modified November 5, 2021, https://www.drugwatch.com/accutane/side-effects/; Kristin Compton, "Accutane Lawsuits," drugwatch, last modified March 25, 2021, https://www.drugwatch.com/accutane/lawsuits/.

25 "Ephedra," National Institutes of Health, https://ods.od.nih.gov/HealthInformation/Ephedra.aspx; Gene Emery, "FDA ban nearly wiped out deaths, poisonings from ephedra," Reuters, May 27, 2015, https://www.reuters.com/article/us-fda-ephedra/fda-ban-nearly-wiped-out-deaths-poisonings-from-ephedra-idUSKBN0OC2SR20150527

Chapter Four

26 National Cancer Institute, "Cancer Stat Facts: Prostate Cancer," National Cancer Institute, last modified 2021, https://seer.cancer.gov/statfacts/html/prost.html.

27 Aaron E. Katz, The Definitive Guide to Prostate Cancer: Everything You Need to Know about Conventional and Integrative Therapies, (Pennsylvania: Rodale, Inc., 2011).

28 Aaron E. Katz, The Definitive Guide to Prostate Cancer: Everything You Need to Know about Conventional and Integrative Therapies, (Pennsylvania: Rodale, Inc., 2011) p. xiii.

Chapter Seven

29 "President Obama Declares September 2010 'National Prostate Cancer Awareness Month,'" PR Newswire, September 1, 2010, https://www.prnewswire.com/news-releases/president-obama-declares-september-2010-national-prostate-cancer-awareness-month-101989848.html.

Chapter Nine

30 E-mail and hard copy of my records from MSKCC.

31 Ian M. Thompson, Donna Pauler Ankerst, Chen Chi, Phyllis J. Good-man, Catherine M. Tangen, Scott M. Lippman, M. Scott Lucia, Howard L. Parnes, and Charles A. Coltman Jr, "Prediction of Prostate Cancer for Patients Receiving Finasteride: Results From the Prostate Cancer Prevention Trial," Journal of Clinical Oncology 25, no. 21 (September 21, 2016), https://ascopubs.org/doi/10.1200/JCO.2006.07.6836.

Chapter Ten

32 Yuval Ramot, Tali Czarnowicki, and Abraham Zlotogorski, "Finasteride induced Gynecomastia: Case report and Review of the Literature," U.S. National Library of Medicine, January 2009, https://www.ncbi.nlm.nih.gov/pmc/articles/PMC2929552/.

33 Muhammad Z U Khan, Shujaat A Khan, Muhammad Ubaid, Aamna Shah, Rozina Kousar, and Ghulam Murtaza, "Finasteride Topical Delivery Systems for Androgenetic Alopecia," National Library of Medicine, 2018, https://pubmed.ncbi.nlm.nih.gov/29366416/; Michelle Llamas, "Chicago Man: 'Taking Propecia is the Biggest Regret of My Life,'" drugwatch, last modified March 4, 2021, https://www.drugwatch.com/beyond-side-effects/chicago-man-taking-propecia-biggest-regret-life/.

34 Ike Swetlitz, "Drugs to combat hair loss could raise risk for erectile dysfunction, study finds," STAT News, March 9, 2017, https://www.statnews.com/2017/03/09/finasteride-erectile-dysfunction/; Ryan Jaslow, "FDA adds sexual sideeffects warning to baldness drug Propecia," CBS News, April 13, 2012, https://www.cbsnews.com/news/fda-adds-sexual-side-effects-warning-to-baldness-drug-propecia/.

35 Dan Levine, "Court let Merck hide secrets about a popular drug's risks," Reuters, September 11, 2019, https://www.reuters.com/investigates/special-report/usa-courts-secrecy-propecia/; Emily Miller, "Propecia

Lawsuits," drugwatch, last modified September 2018, https://www. drugwatch.com/propecia/lawsuits/.

36 Dan Levine, "Court let Merck hide secrets about a popular drug's risks," Reuters, September 11, 2019, https://www.reuters.com/investigates/special-report/usa-courts-secrecy-propecia/; Emily Miller, "Propecia Lawsuits," drugwatch, last modified September 2018, https://www.drugwatch. com/propecia/lawsuits/.

Chapter Eleven

37 Jessica Ryen Doyle, "Prostate Cancer: 'Not Just an Old Man's Cancer,'" FOX News, last modified October 24, 2015, https://www.foxnews.com/ health/prostate-cancer-not-just-an-old-mans-cancer.

38 "Who We Are," Cancer Schmancer, https://www.cancerschmancer.org/ who-we-are.

Chapter Thirteen

39 Rahim Kanani, "How Facebook is Changing the World for Good," Forbes, May 29, 2012, http://www.forbes.com/sites/rahimkanani/2012/05/29/how-facebook-is-changing-the-world-for-good/.

40 "Treatment Tips: Planning and Preparing," American Institute for Cancer Research, https://www.aicr.org/cancer-survival/treatment-tips/during-treatment/ #1579143237677-fe3251cd-d744.

41 TEDx Talks, "Changing the way we fight cancer: Gabe Canales at TEDx-Houston 2013," YouTube, 16:13, October 29, 2013, https://youtu.be/ rm7UpHIqWmg.

42 National Cancer Institute, "Prostate-Specific Antigen (PSA) Test," National Cancer Institute, last modified 2021, https://www.cancer.gov/ types/prostate/psa-fact-sheet.

43 National Cancer Institute, "Cancer Stat Facts: Prostate Cancer," National Cancer Institute, last modified 2021, https://seer.cancer.gov/statfacts/ html/prost.html.

Chapter Fourteen

44 LaSalle D. Lefall, Jr. and Margaret L. Kripke, "2008–2009 Annual Report, President's Cancer Panel: REDUCING ENVIRONMENTAL CANCER RISK, What We Can Do Now," National Institutes of Health, 2009, https://deainfo.nci.nih.gov/advisory/pcp/annualreports/pcp08-09rpt/pcp_report_08-09_508.pdf.

45 Margaret I. Cuomo, "Are We Wasting Billions Seeking a Cure for Cancer?" Daily Beast, last modified July 14, 2017, https://www.thedailybeast.com/are-we-wasting-billions-seeking-a-cure-for-cancer.

46 Margaret I. Cuomo, A World without Cancer: The Making of a New Cure and the Real Promise of Prevention (Pennsylvania: Rodale, Inc, 2013).

47 LaSalle D. Lefall, Jr. and Margaret L. Kripke, "2008–2009 Annual Report, President's Cancer Panel: REDUCING ENVIRONMENTAL CANCER RISK, What We Can Do Now," National Institutes of Health, 2009, https://deainfo.nci.nih.gov/advisory/pcp/annualreports/pcp08-09rpt/pcp_report_08-09_508.pdf.

Chapter Fifteen

48 "7,800 mile road trip raising awareness for men's health," FOX 26 Houston, May 23, 2019, https://www.fox26houston.com/houstons-morning-show/7800-mile-road-trip-raising-awareness-for-mens-health.

49 Epidemiology and Public Health Preparedness, "Austin Public Health: Critical Health Indicators Report 2017," The City of Austin, Texas, March 20, 2017, https://www.austintexas.gov/sites/default/files/files/Health/Epidemiology/CHI_Report_3.20.17.pdf; "Deaths By Suicide And Suicide Attempts In Austin-Travis County," Corridor News, August 18, 2018, https://smcorridornews.com/deaths-by-suicide-and-suicide-attempts-in-austin-travis-county/.

50 "Overweight & Obesity in Bexar County," City of San Antonio Metropolitan Health District, 2014, https://www.sanantonio.gov/Portals/0/Files/health/HealthyLiving/FactSheet-Obesity-English.pdf

51 "2017 Annual Sexually Transmitted Disease Surveillance Report," Los Angeles County Department of Public Health, September 9, 2018, http://www.publichealth.lacounty.gov/dhsp/Reports/STD/2017_STDSurveillanceReport_Final_07.29.19.pdf.

52 American Cancer Society, "New Mexico At A Glance," American Cancer Society, last modified 2021, https://cancerstatisticscenter.cancer.org/#!/state/New%20Mexico.

53 American Cancer Society, "Washington At A Glance," American Cancer Society, last modified 2021, https://cancerstatisticscenter.cancer.org/#!/state/Washington.

54 "King County Medical Examiner's Office Annual Report 2017," Public Health Seattle & King County, 2017, https://kingcounty.gov/depts/health/examiner/~/media/depts/health/medical-examiner/documents/King-County-Medical-Examiner-2017-Annual-Report.ashx.

55 American Cancer Society, "Utah At A Glance," American Cancer Society, last modified 2021, https://cancerstatisticscenter.cancer.org/#!/state/Utah.

56 Tobacco Prevention and Cessation Commission, "Indiana Adult Smoking," Indiana.gov, February 25, 2020, https://www.in.gov/health/tpc/files/IN-Adult-Smoking_02_25_2020.pdf; "Overweight & Obesity, Data & Statistics," Centers for Disease Control and Prevention, last modified November 10, 2021, https://www.cdc.gov/obesity/data/index.html; Craig M. Hales, Margaret D. Carroll, Cheryl D. Fryar, and Cynthia L. Ogden, "Prevalence of Obesity and Severe Obesity Among Adults: United States, 2017–2018," Centers for Disease Control and Prevention, last modified February 27, 2020, https://www.cdc.gov/nchs/products/databriefs/db360.htm.

57 "Overweight & Obesity, Data & Statistics," Centers for Disease Control and Prevention, last modified November 10, 2021, https://www.cdc.gov/obesity/data/index.html.

58 American Cancer Society, "New York At A Glance," American Cancer Society, last modified 2021, https://cancerstatisticscenter.cancer.org/#!/state/New%20York.

59 "Cancer Statistics," National Cancer Institute, last modified September 25, 2020, https://www.cancer.gov/about-cancer/understanding/statistics.

60 "Men and Heart Disease," Centers for Disease Control and Prevention, last modified February 3, 2021, https://www.cdc.gov/heartdisease/men.htm.

61 "Overweight & Obesity Statistics," National Institute of Diabetes and Digestive and Kidney Diseases, last modified August 2017, https://www.

niddk.nih.gov/health-information/health-statistics/overweight-obesity; "Overweight & Obesity: Why It Matters," Centers for Disease Control and Prevention, last modified March 1, 2021, https://www.cdc.gov/obesity/about-obesity/why-it-matters.html; Sharon Begley, "Fat and getting fatter: U.S. obesity rates to soar by 2030," Reuters, September 18, 2012, https://www.reuters.com/article/us-obesity-us/fat-and-getting-fatter-u-s-obesity-rates-to-soar-by-2030-idUSBRE88H0RA20120918.

[62] "Overweight & Obesity, Data & Statistics," Centers for Disease Control and Prevention, last modified November 10, 2021, https://www.cdc.gov/obesity/data/index.html.

[63] "Overweight & Obesity, Data & Statistics," Centers for Disease Control and Prevention, last modified November 10, 2021, https://www.cdc.gov/obesity/data/index.html.

[64] "Lung Cancer Fact Sheet: Smoking-Attributable Lung Cancer," American Lung Association, last modified May 27, 2020, https://www.lung.org/lung-health-diseases/lung-disease-lookup/lung-cancer/resource-library/lung-cancer-fact-sheet.

[65] "Adult Obesity Causes & Consequences," Centers for Disease Control and Prevention, last modified March 22, 2021, https://www.cdc.gov/obesity/adult/causes.html.

[66] "Obesity and Cancer," Centers for Disease Control and Prevention, last modified February 18, 2021, https://www.cdc.gov/cancer/obesity/index.htm.

[67] "What are the Lifestyle-Related Risk Factors for Prostate Cancer?: Weight," American Institute for Cancer Research, last modified November 10, 2020, https://www.aicr.org/cancer-survival/cancer/prostate-cancer/.

Chapter Sixteen

[68] "Overweight & Obesity Statistics," National Institute of Diabetes and Digestive and Kidney Diseases, last modified August 2017, https://www.niddk.nih.gov/health-information/health-statistics/overweight-obesity.

[69] Jessica Ryen Doyle, "Prostate Cancer: 'Not Just an Old Man's Cancer,'" FOX News, last modified October 24, 2015, https://www.foxnews.com/health/prostate-cancer-not-just-an-old-mans-cancer.

70 "Best Heart-Healthy Diets," U.S. News & World Report, https://health. usnews.com/best-diet/best-heart-healthy-diets.

71 Anders Anglesey, "World's COVID Deaths Reach 5 Million, With More in U.S. Than Anywhere Else," Newsweek, November 1, 2021, https:// www.newsweek.com/world-covid-deaths-5million-united-states-leads-country-fatalities-1644450; Kristen Monaco, " Over 73% of U.S. Adults Overweight or Obese," Medpage Today, December 11, 2020, https:// www.medpagetoday.com/primarycare/obesity/90142; "Chronic Diseases in America," Centers for Disease Control and Prevention, last modified January 12, 2021, https://www.cdc.gov/chronicdisease/resources/ infographic/chronic-diseases.htm; Berkeley Lovelace Jr, "CDC study finds about 78% of people hospitalized for Covid were overweight or obese," CNBC, last modified March 9, 2021, https://www.cnbc. com/2021/03/08/covid-cdc-study-finds-roughly-78percent-of-people-hospitalized-were-overweight-or-obese.html

72 Office on Women's Health, "Creation of Offices on Women's Health at the federal level," U.S. Department of Health & Human Services, last modified April 1, 2019, https://www.womenshealth.gov/30-achievements/17.

ACKNOWLEDGMENTS

This book would not be possible without the support of the Blue Cure community and the tens of thousands of prostate cancer patients, caregivers, patient advocates, and medical professionals I have met since my diagnosis in 2010. Thank you for sharing your experiences, insights, challenges, and hopes. You have taught me immensely and I am incredibly grateful.

I extend my heartfelt thanks to the numerous individuals who have impacted me in various ways throughout my journey with prostate cancer. Your words and actions (no matter how small), served as inspiration and motivation in my advocacy and efforts to share, educate, inform, and move men to act. Thank you Elizabeth and Glenn Howard, my dad, Carl and Sue Rowold, Chad and Geni Gonsoulin, Jim McClellan, Carolyn Farb, Sofia van der Dys, Tristan van der Dys, Alexa van der Dys, Chris and Jenny Myers, Dr. Rod Paige, Ryan Pontbriand, Dustin Roy, Ethan Etzel, Craig Steinfeld, AJ and Siobahn Gracely, Sherry Eichberger, Vern Montross, Carlos Perez, Jenny Johnson, Mynette Murtagh, James Munisteri, John Mendelsohn, MD, Lorenzo Cohen, PhD, Larry Lipshultz, MD, Peter Pinto, MD, Dean Ornish, MD, Aaron Katz, MD, Jonathan Haas, MD, Philippa Cheetham, MD, Ashutosh Tewari, MD, Ketan Badani, MD, Margaret I. Cuomo, MD, Geo Espinosa, ND, John N. Papadopoulos, MD, Shalin Shah, MD, Alex Pastuszak, MD, PhD, Tomasz M. Beer, MD, Charles Modlin, MD, Lily Jang, Dale Lockett, Deborah Duncan, Dominique Sachse, Chita Craft, Vicente Arenas, Lucy Noland, Alex Sanz, Frank Billingsley, Ryan Chase, Alex Cadelago, 104.1 KRBE, Meghan O' Hara, Keith Klein, Brittany Zucker, Winell Heron, H-E-B, Kristina Leal Jewasko, Jana and

Richard Fant, Wallis and DeeDee Marsh, Barbara and Peter Forbes, Jimmy Montgomery, Conor Grier, Donald Kilgore, John Garza, Paul-David Van Atta, Jackie Medina, Barry Cik, Naturepedic, David Bentkowski, Liz Anklow, Pete Olson, Ed Brown, Diana Turner, Dee Koch, Former Mayor Annise Parker, Mayor Sylvester Turner, Sheriff Ed Gonzalez, Laura Pettitt, Bruce Westbrook, Nick Colvin, Andy Rowold, Debra Moyer, Todd Smith, Anthony Medina, University of St. Thomas, UST Athletics, Stephanie Tarbox-Kerns, Eric Mendez, Fran Drescher, Cancer Schmancer, Susan Cassel-Holland, Hope Smith, Bob Saget, Matt Schaub, Erin Brockovich, John Mackey, Sir Roger Moore, Lady Kristina.

I express my gratitude to those directly involved in making this book possible: Austin Miller, Martha Miller, Dupree Miller & Associates, Heather King, Debra Englander and the team at Post Hill Press, Tom Zenner, Grant Denham.

ABOUT THE AUTHOR

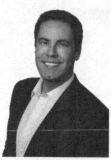

AUTHOR PHOTO: SOFIA VAN DER DYS

Gabe Canales serves as the powerhouse behind the Blue Cure Foundation, the force behind several high-impact national campaigns and a social media community for men's health with over 200,000 followers, including athletes and celebrities.

For the last decade, Canales has been a leading voice in men's health advocacy on the national stage. Canales has been featured in *Forbes,* as a TEDx speaker, and has served as served as a panelist for the American Association of Cancer Researchers and the Society of Nuclear Medicine Conference. He has also been a keynote speaker for groups like the Oregon Urology Association and the Indian American Cancer Network, along with serving as emcee for MD Anderson Cancer Center's Ride of a Lifetime. Canales has contributed to the *Houston Chronicle* and *The Huffington Post,* along with appearing in numerous media outlets throughout the country.

In 2019, Canales embarked on a forty-city media tour, driving 8,867 miles on a road trip throughout the United States, bringing awareness to the most pressing men's health issues in each region. His goal was to inspire men to take action and own their health outcomes. Along the way, the meaningful conversations he had with doctors, researchers, survivors, health experts, journalists and thought leaders led to the decision to write a book to share the knowledge he gained.